Fancy All That

by

Penny Fell

© Penny Fell

'Looking Glass' series published by:

Pipers' Ash World Wide

www.supamasu.com

CHIPPENHAM   WILTSHIRE   ENGLAND

SN15 4BW

Dedicated to Andrew,
family and friends, who are
the best medicines

'Gloucester Edition'
ISBN 9781904494973

Chapters

1 *My Young Life*

MY YOUNG LIFE was quite eventful. I was and still am accident prone and was always getting into scrapes. Life was fun and for adventures and I enjoyed it.

When I was 10 years old I went to Guide camp, but wasn't there long as I had a 'black out'. They were very polite in the 60's and didn't call them fits.

Not long after this my life fell apart as my Mum and Dad divorced and it was hard to cope with being in the middle, but I plodded along having the odd black out on the way.

I was a very lanky athletic teenager who loved swimming and walking. I threw myself into school and got into Waverley College in Nottingham to do Nursery Nursing.

I left home at 16 years old and was living in a bed-sit in Nottingham and my boyfriend Andy wanted to go to the cinema to see the new James Bond Movie. We didn't see much as I had a bad fit and a man in the audience came over and said; 'She has epilepsy, I will drive you home'. Andy's Mum Dot took care of me and I lived there for a while as the stress of living of my own, college work and a few part time jobs was getting too much for me. In those days, early 70's, I received a wage of £8 a week from college as we worked in Nurseries /schools 3 days a week. I had to have 2 part time jobs to pay for the books etc.

I went to the Doctors and after many hospital visits and tests; I was diagnosed as an epileptic. My specialist was Dr Whiteley and I can remember the day when I sat in front of him and he told me what I couldn't do any more. I couldn't drive. This was a great blow as for the last 2 years all I had thought about was passing my driving test and buying a mini car. Then he said to 'avoid' discos.

'Stuff that', I thought, here was me only 17 years old and being told to keep out of discos! I learnt very quickly to dance with your eyes looking down or shut. This was a big disadvantage if you wanted to look lovingly into your fellas eyes, but Andy was very understanding.

The next thing I was told too avoid was sex and I wouldn't be able to have children. I was distraught; what no sex! I had just discovered it! Apparently too much excitement could trigger a fit. A bit embarrassing and uncomfortable for your man if this happened in the middle of nookie! Also I had been told not go to the cinema. My trigger was flashing lights and they still bother me now (30 odd years later).

After bawling my eyes out for two days and feeling very sorry for myself, I decided too get on with life.

This was the start of a life long struggle to make people realise that I am me and not a word in a textbook.

The fact that I was training to be a Nursery Nurse, but now was an epileptic led to me being called into the heads office at college. I had just finished the first year of a two year course. Unbelievably the Head decided that I was a good student and that if I changed tactics and didn't work with babies and under two's I could carry on training! I owe a lot to that woman.

Life was looking good again!

I was put on Phenobarbitone, (now banned) which are very funny tablets. At first I just wanted to sleep all the time which was unusual for me as I am hyper active and my mind never stops.

My philosophy of my life was that if I am not allowed to do something then try a little bit and if I didn't fit, then carry on. This is how things like sex, going to the pictures, discos and even riding a bike (not on really busy streets!) crept back into my life. After a while you get used to the warning signals and having a bad day. This was the days when your body temperature just dropped, you felt sick, the room kept going around and you just wanted to crawl under a blanket on the settee. I usually couldn't get my words out and it sounded like I was drunk. There were no help groups out there then and you didn't tell people that you were an epileptic or else they thought you were mad and needed to be put into a mental hospital.

One of the main side effects from taking pheno's was my weight. Now I was 5ft 8inches tall and was quite slimish. My weight went up from 9 stones right up to 10 and a half stones in a couple of weeks! This has been the bane of my life, my weight and trying to lose it. I didn't realise it then but my tables had a sort of steroid in them which caused this. I wasn't a huge eater and didn't like meat much.

Anyway I passed college and Andy and I got married. My hubby is great. He is my friend as well as my husband and without him I wouldn't be here writing this story. When you think what he has put up with he deserves a medal. I thought he would run away after seeing me in the cinema that night, but no, he has looked after me and made me feel 'normal'.

2 Coping with Life

WE MANAGED to get a mortgage. I was working in a great school and Andy was Hairdressing. When I was feeling 'off' at school the teacher whose class I was in noticed that I had gone pale and my eyes would dim and she would take me to the staff room. Sometimes I had to come home, but not very often. I was happy there and usually if you are happy you don't have a fit. Now I have two types of fits. They call them different names nowadays, but I have always known them as Petit Malls (petit) or Grand Malls (biggy). The petit's are where you just freeze and your eyes roll to the back of your head and then you come out of it. These affect me in several ways; sometimes I come out of them and feel ok. In fact if I am playing monopoly or something I find my houses have suddenly disappeared! (We tend to treat my disability with a laugh, it's the ONLY way I can get through life, but that's me!). Then if it goes on longer for a couple of minutes I end up disorientated and a have major pain in my head. It's quite weird if I am on the phone, I have to put my hand over it and ask Andy what I was talking about! Or if I am talking to someone at the time. I think a lot of people must think I am a bit barking. My knees get bashed and sometimes broken, this is a downer. If you are standing, whomph, down you go on the old knees! I am always covered in bruises.

Grand Malls are something else; luckily for me I usually have them at night. I don't know why, maybe it's because when I am lying there in bed my mind starts worrying about things. Now epileptics don't just writhe and shake all over on the floor, it seems as if an Alien has taken over your body and it gets bashed about unmercifully. Then the next stage starts, I call my yucky stage, where your stomach and bowels do not belong to you and decide to empty themselves. This can be verrrrrrrrry embarrassing. Luckily I cannot remember who I am, where I am, what date it is, nothing. So I am unaware what I have done for a while. Andy has cleaned up after me and never complained. Sometimes he tells me afterwards if I have 'been' in odd places, like once I got up out of bed, had a fit, and then went to the toilet in the linen chest on top of all the clean ironed sheets! You have got to laugh at these things or you would curl up and die.

I got used to this life and tried to pretend it was another me.

Now the Specialist at Queens Medical Hospital told me that I wouldn't be able to have children, but my doctor advised me to got on the birth pill, just in case. They also found a patch on my brain, which was like a bruise. This might have been caused in the four years that I lived in a Children's hostel from the age of 11 years to 15 years and they believed in punishments, such as the hairbrush on the bare bottom and such. I also got beaten up a bit, but don't dwell on those years as I want to forget them.

New house new baby and you've guessed I fell pregnant. What I or the doctor didn't realise was that if you are taking pheno's the pill is cancelled out! We now know.

My pregnancy took its toll on me. I would come home from work and go to sleep on the settee. Andy was doing all the housework. I was in and out of hospital for bed rest and by now Andy had finished Hairdressing as he knew he couldn't make enough to support a family (which we really wanted) and was working for Boots in the warehouse on Island Street. He loved working there and they were very understanding. He would phone me whenever he had a break.

I finished work at the Christmas and Kirsti was born on February 12th 1977.

She was our little miracle, as I had died during birth after too many fits, but I wasn't ready to give up and I starting breathing again as she was born.

Life with a baby was different and being an epileptic with a baby was even more different. I didn't want to have a fit and hurt my baby, so made sure that when picking her up I didn't walk far with her in my arms unless someone was with me. I loved having a daughter to sit and cuddle and realised this is what I had always wanted in life, a family.

I was worried that Kirsti would be like me and the doctors said that if she hadn't had a fit by the time she was 3 years old, then she should be ok. Mine wasn't heredity. The only thing she couldn't have was certain immunisation jabs (like the measles one). I also breast fed and was worried that my tablets would be passed on to her, but they dismissed this and I carried on. Now, if I sleep I usually feel better if I am having/had a bad day and during feeding at night I would usually drop off! Andy would wake up and put Kirsti in her cot when she had finished. It became instinct.

I was warned not to have any more children and I went on all sorts of birth control devises, some too weird to recall. The birth foam was funny though! Anyway, I fell pregnant again 6 months after having Kirsti and the Doctors wanted to terminate the baby. I refused and struggled through another pregnancy. This time wasn't too bad as I wasn't working and could rest more. I remember being told to drink Guinness as my iron count was low! I did this with both pregnancies and I am not very good with alcohol as it makes me drunk very quickly, so this was really bizarre. They wouldn't suggest it nowadays! My teeth and gums suffered during pregnancy. I often woke in the morning with my tongue split as I had had a fit in the night. Sometimes it would be a 'small' grand mal for a few seconds, so I woke feeling groggy and sore. I now have problems drinking hot or very cold drinks or food because of my battered tongue.

Ross was born on 11th October 1978 and I saw him being born this time. I was still in and out of it but we both survived. My second miracle, but my last as the Doctor asked Andy if they could sterilise me and he agreed. He daren't tell me and the day after the birth I was in the operating theatre again. I was upset but relieved.

Having two children was exhausting but I loved it. They got used to Mummy's funny turns; luckily I never had a biggy in front of them until they were older. Now I was still on pheno's and taking more when I had bad days. I could have taken even more and had no fits but would have lived in a constant haze and didn't want that. So I had a few petits a week and a biggy every month or so.

3 Trying to Get A Job

IN 1979, trying to get a job when you had a disability wasn't easy, so you kept quiet and hoped for the best. Nobody would employ me as a Nursery Nurse.

So I went around the local Business's. That's how I got a job as a cleaner at the Glass factory. Now glass and epileptics don't usually go hand in hand and when I walked into the showroom and saw all the glass shelves and shiny floor I thought' 'Oh flipping heck'. My job was to clean the offices and shine that nice floor with the huge polisher on Wednesday and Friday nights. So Andy when came home and I went out. I loved it and that polisher was something, you could actually stand on the back of it and ride it! Then a few months later I had a fit at work and got the sack instantaneously. I didn't break anything though. My next job was a glass washer (glass again!) behind a bar in a large hotel near Clarendon college. I learnt how to be a barmaid and enjoyed it, but after a couple of weeks a new law came in. All employees had to have a medical. So the next evening I went to work and the Doctor was there giving medicals to all the staff. Guess who the doctor was? Yep, mine! I was sacked. So I went on the job hunt again and my friend told me of a bar job going in Sherwood Rooms which was a place that held Discos, cabarets, shows and allsorts of venues.

It was in Nottingham, so I had to get the bus there for the interview and I got the job. I loved it and worked with some great people. My Boss was very firm but a good man. I worked on Friday and Saturday nights to begin with and I got a taxi there and they paid for our taxi's home. It was long hours, sometimes not getting home until 2 am. Then I had a fit but didn't get the sack. The Boss was cross because I hadn't told him the truth, but I said 'would you have given me the job? Basically I have worked hard and could prove that I could do the job'. He agreed with that and kept me on. If I had a fit then they dragged me into the storeroom! Luckily I didn't have many at work. My hours lengthened and I was working 4 to 5 nights a week and sometimes the odd Saturday at Trent Bridge Cricket Club at a bar in the Marquee. If you worked Christmas Eve, Boxing night and New Years Eve you got treble time cash in hand, so I did those as well. My wages paid for holidays and other luxuries, like fitted carpets!

Kirsti and Ross were used to having a nap with Mum in the afternoons when we all went to sleep on the settee! When they started Nursery, I would get up take them there, come home, have breakfast and go back to bed with the alarm on. This is the way I coped.

One Christmas I was sitting on the loo and had a big attack causing me to fall off and break my nose and the loo roll holder (from habitat, no less!). I ended up in hospital and that Christmas had two huge plaster things across my nose and two black eyes. I was really mad that I had broken the loo holder!

So I cut my hours down a bit, money is good, but not everything.

I worked there until 1982, and in the same year had the worst fit since giving birth.

It was just after the New Year and I had worked all over the holidays. The children, Kirsti was 5 years old (now at school) and Ross 3 years old were in bed asleep and I went to have a bath. Now Andy sometimes used to sit with me or he kept an ear out, good job really as he heard a thump, then silence and he ran upstairs.

I was having a fit and was under the water.

What had happened was that I was soaking and wanted more hot water, so I turned the tap on with my foot. Our water tank had just been on and the water was boiling, literally, (the thermostat had broken and we didn't know).

13

It burnt my foot and the pain caused me to have a fit. As I was 'out of it', the water burnt my legs, feet and my groin. Andy pulled me up and took the plug out, but I had already knocked it out and the soap had melted and clogged up the plug hole as the water was so hot, burning his hand as he did so. Everything that happened from then on was hazy; all I remember is coming around in the hospital and a big Nurse looming over me popping the blisters on the bottom of my feet and ankles. The Sister came over and asked her what she was doing. She was furious and told the nurse off. Then they wrapped me in gooey stuff and I zonked out.

I was sent home in an ambulance as there were no spare beds.

Andy took the children to school and Nursery the next morning, and then he had to nip into work to talk to his boss to get some time off. He told me to stay in bed and not move.

I couldn't and was living from one painkiller to the next one. I was woken up by someone knocking on our front door. Now we slept on two mattresses as these were nearer to the floor and if I had a fit in the night it wasn't too far to fall, so I eased myself out of bed and shuffled on my bottom to the stairs. They kept knocking on the door and I shouted to say I was coming. Then I tried to get down the stairs and fell all the way down. I knocked myself out.

Andy came home and found me and phoned the ambulance. I had broken my left leg in several places, both knees and my right ankle. So I had a plaster cast on each leg right up to my crutch which was covered in blisters. I was told to rest and not move for at least a month! Arrgh! It was agony. Andy made me a bed up on the settee and asked me to be good.

I couldn't move if I wanted to. I had to go to the loo in a bowl! Andy only got a week off work, and then my friend who lived next door would come around and take the children to school and collect them. The children were really good and got used to not sitting on my legs. Kirsti had a little pot tea set and loved plating tea parties with me, I drank loads of little cups of yucky water and saying; 'Yum that's lovely!' She was Mummy.

They would lie besides me and loved watching the television and playing games and things. Andy would get them ready in the morning and he would leave me sandwiches and a drink and anything else I would need next to me. I couldn't have got through the ordeal without him and friends and family who would come and see me. The phone bill soared! I was so bored though. I was still on painkillers so slept a lot when the children weren't there. I really missed a proper wash, not one in a bowl!

The Doctor kept visiting me and explained that I would be scarred where the blisters were popped and the ones on my crutch were healing quite well. The soles of my feet are now very sensitive. I didn't have a fit for ages, maybe it's because I was on another planet on painkillers! Andy would sometimes make a bed on the floor besides me and sleep with me, holding my hand.

I could feel myself getting fatter as I wasn't allowed to move or exercise.

At the end of the month I was looking forward to the plasters coming off, but when I went to hospital they only took the left one off. My right leg wasn't healing properly.

It was bliss getting one off, I could wash it! I still wasn't allowed upstairs and had to sit with my leg up again for another month. I missed my life and felt very guilty with Andy doing everything, he was so tired.

It was nearly 3 months before the other cast came off and I had to learn to walk again with a Zimmer frame and then a stick. My leg was really white and skinny!

I had had 3 months off work and they kept my job open.

After a couple of weeks building my muscles up I started working one night a week then gradually more.

Then we were all made redundant and they shut the Sherwood Rooms down.

So I was without a job again. I started looking after a couple of children who I collected with my own from Nursery and then their Mum would come around for them after she had finished work. I didn't earn much but they were no trouble and I love kids so it was easy. We had found out at this time that Kirsti was partially deaf and we were taking her for tests. She eventually had a hearing aid which helped, but she preferred not to wear it as 'everything was too loud'! She could lip read and we are a noisy family anyway so that helps!

The pub up the street had a vacancy for Friday and Saturday nights so I went for the job and got it. The landlord and lady were great and I really enjoyed working for them. I told them about me and if I had a fit then they would phone Andy and he came and fetched me home. This worked quite well and luckily it didn't happen a lot, then my luck changed and I had a fit when the Brewery Boss came in and he sacked me on the spot.

The Landlord was furious with them and he would often phone me if it was a busy night, so no worries.

I had managed to lose a little weight gained when I was in plaster cast and I now was about 11 stones.

I can remember going vegetarian as I had never eaten a lot of meat any way, but when I visited Dr Whitely (My visits had gone down to one a year and they left me alone as they didn't really know what to do with me) he told me off and said I needed to eat meat as this might stop me having so many fits. I needed the nourishment or something. I was flummoxed, but I wasn't the expert so I started eating chicken. It didn't make much difference. He also told me to stop working or I would end up in a wheelchair by the time I was 50 years old (I am 52 now and still walking!) and most probably wouldn't see 60 years. This made me a bit down, but I resolved to prove him wrong!

In 1983, with our insurance money we went on holiday to Norway. My Dad came with us and he drove, as I am not allowed and Andy only drove a motorbike.

It changed our lives and opened our eyes to all the beautiful countryside in this world.

I was calm and fine all holiday. When we were there we asked about getting jobs there and emigrating, but found out that because we have the N.H.S. in Britain, my tablets there would cost nearly all our wages a week. Also they wanted healthy people there with no disabilities.

Soon after this we decided that we had had enough of the City and moved to the country.

4 Underwood

It Was Brilliant in Underwood, a different way of life and we were surrounded by countryside. I was happy getting the house straight and I had a large garden for growing vegetables in, bliss! This was our kind of life. We had a coal fire so the time was spent with chopping wood and just getting on with life and I felt a different person. I was calmer.

I kept quiet about being an epileptic and when I took the children to school, which was just around the corner, I kept my mouth shut. The children loved their new school and at weekends we all packed a picnic and walked for miles, there was plenty to discover.

Andy went to and from work on his motor bike and we were used to travelling around on buses, trains and sometimes with friends. Despite being an epileptic, I was generally quite healthy and walked for miles, though my knees were beginning to give me grief. Also my tummy had been playing me up for years and I just put it down to side effects with my tablets. I wasn't very good at eating processed foods, but I liked baking and cooking, so no problem. If I put too much weight on I went on Slim Fast for a couple of weeks, but they made me really bad and I was on the loo a lot. I suppose that's how I lost the weight! I often just ate fruit and veg but I never lost any weight. I had to watch pastry and cakes though; I could put 3 pounds on in one day with them!

Getting a job was harder in a village than in the city. I helped my next door neighbour clean at the local miner's welfare club.

I was having petits but I hadn't had a biggy for ages until one day I felt really rough. So I walked up the road to a woman's house because she had always talked to me at school. I just needed to talk to someone and I might feel better. She opened the door and I said hello, are you alright'? She looked at me asked if I was drunk and slammed the door in my face. I staggered home and had a fit on the driveway and my knees slammed into the concrete. Someone saw me and picked me up and took me indoors. They became good friends. I made more friends in the village and told them the truth about me. They accepted it. People were getting better at seeing me as a person and not a mad woman! That reminds me of when I was about 17yrs old and I had a lot of biggy's then, well I had one in Nottingham Market Square and I remember the ambulance, then coming to on a bed. There were two doctors/nurses looking at me. The man said; 'She's drunk', but the woman said; 'No she's not, I think she's had a fit' Then she asked me to stick out my tongue which was chewed again and nodded her head. It's amazing on how many people have thought I was a drunk!

After the New Year in 1986 I started having problems with my periods and had a lot of tummy pains. Now it had been like this for years, but not as bad and my other doctor said it was indigestion, so I didn't worry and thought this was normal. I went to my new Doctor; he took one look at my tummy and made an appointment at the City Hospital for the next week.

Andy took the day off and came with me. I sat there and the specialist said; 'If you don't stop smoking you will be dead within a year!' I was speechless I hardly smoked any more. I had smoked off and on since I was 15, more when I worked behind the bar, but that was due to stress. I only had about one a day now if that. I never smoked in front of Andy or the children and he just glared at me!

The doctor said I had to stay in for a couple of days as he wanted to run tests on me. I was admitted that afternoon and Andy went home to pack me a bag and sort the children out with a babysitter.

I had tests and I had cancer of the womb. I had to have a full hysterectomy immediately.

The operation was very long and I had a big fit in the middle, but I was ok. I remember waking up and talking to a Nurse and wanting to pee like a horse. They fetched a commode and helped me out of bed. I got back in and I had a relapse, my stitches burst.

I passed out.

I ended up back in the operating theatre. It was very hazy and I had had enough so I gave up. I remember floating among white stuff and hearing Andy crying; 'Don't leave me Pen'. That's when I started breathing again, life was good. I was only 31 years old!

I was in hospital for nearly 6 weeks. Whilst I was in there a social worker came to visit me. She was surprised that I had never had anybody visit me before. The first thing she did was sort out my tablets, as they were a barbiturate and had been banned. The doctor decided to put me onto Epilum. I nicknamed this the weight tablet, 'cos that's what they do! I had stopped smoking too so that didn't help and I soared up to 14 stones from 11 stones in 6 weeks! She asked me what disability payments I was on and I was gob smacked, what disability payments? She was surprised and brought me papers to fill in. I had a health card too and when I looked on it, it said; Penelope Sue Fell; Incurable.

I thought Charming! Andy looked at it and laughed and said I was Incorrigible! So we treated it as a joke and it didn't seem so bad.

I loved it when Andy and the children visited me; they were like a breath of fresh air.

There was this really posh woman who came in for an operation with equally posh husband and awful children. She didn't talk much even though I tried to be nice. One day after visiting hours she looked up and asked; Are you here for the same as me?' I asked what she had done and she said with no embarrassment; 'Oh, a fanny tuck darling' I didn't know whether to laugh or say; 'you what!?!' I just sat there and went; 'Oh, well that's nice, no I haven't' I couldn't believe that she told me. It takes all sorts!

I had to take life slowly after this, but at least we were financially better off thanks to my Fairy Godmother. After a few months I went to see Dr Whitely and he took me off Epilum and onto Tegretol 200mg, I have 4 to 5 a day. They gave me a new lease of life!

He also said he didn't need to see me again as he couldn't help me any more. I was to go to my Doctor instead.

Now in 1983 there wasn't a lot of after care and the blood wasn't checked for aids. Luckily I am fine and didn't dwell on it.

After the op I was distraught and didn't feel like a woman as I wanted lots of children. I know this was not possible and I felt lucky to have two. It was just a feeling.

Life got back to normal, well our kind of normal, and then Andy was in a road accident. He was on the way to work on his motor bike and a sports car came out of Maws lane, Kimberley, and smashed straight into him, trapping him under the car.

I wondered if we had moved to the wrong village as since we had been there both of us have been in hospital! It was me this time worrying about Andy and he was in hospital for about 5 weeks. He was smashed up quite badly, thank goodness for his leathers and crash helmet. Without those I wouldn't have a husband now. The worst thing was the bottom of his left leg; it was fixed together inside by titanium steel 'ladder'. He caught the hospital bug from this which led to over 14 operations on his leg and him losing his job, but not his leg. He is now in constant pain.

Later on we discovered acupuncture which relieves this a little. Boots were very good to us at the beginning, but sick pay doesn't last for ever. We were both now classed as disabled. Andy was in a wheelchair on and off for years until his leg grew stronger. He now walks with a stick and has good days and bad. Painkillers help a little and determination.

Because of lifting Andy my stomach got a bit strained which didn't help it.

We moved our bedroom downstairs into the 'playroom' as the bathroom was down there and it made life easier.

The kids weren't very happy about losing their snooker table though! Kirsti had our big bedroom so she was happy about that.

Life carried on, but now we were both unemployable.

5 Wishes & New Beginnings

B Y THE MIDDLE of 1987 we realised that Andy would never go back to work at Boots. So we needed to earn some money somehow to pay the mortgage as the amount we had from disability didn't help with this. If we lived in rented property you had help with it, but no help if the house was your own. Luckily we grew our own veg and I baked so that helped. I can remember going through a phase of eating baked potatoes because that's all we could afford. So we moved Kirsti into the small bedroom and rented out the big one for a while. This kept us from losing the house. It had its problems, but what can you do when you had the bailiffs sniffing around?

Besides the financial problems we were and are a close happy family, I mean nobody lives without the odd argument, but we coped. I had the odd fit here and there, but by now they were part of my life, so I just got on with it.

My disability affected our son, now nearly 10 yrs old as he was at that stage in life where other children would tease him about his Mum and Dad. He would often come home from school with an enormous bruise and a chip on his shoulder. He brushed it off as he didn't want to hurt me with the details. His friends found out that I was an epileptic on the day I decided to knock the chimney out in our sitting room. I was throwing the bricks into a wheelbarrow. Now Andy was unable to help, but the kids helped and things were going really well until I pushed the wheelbarrow to the side of the house. It was too heavy which caused me to have a fit in front of my son's friends. He was traumatised.

So was I when I found out my children protected me as much as I protected them. Bricks give you strange bruises though; you could read them on my legs!

Then our luck began to change.

We had received a bit of money from Andy's written off motor bike and I wanted to use it for something useful and that would cheer Andy up, so we bought a portable Darkroom kit. This became a godsend to me as it keep Andy's mind occupied and he found a hidden talent; photography and developing photographs.

The only downside was that my kitchen became a part time darkroom! This became rather annoying but at least Andy had something to do with his life and he could develop photos whilst in his wheelchair. (He could walk around a little by now, but not a lot).

It was about this time that I decided that I would like to help children with the same disabilities as me. By now, a few more people knew what I was in the village and accepted me, which was great. Every so often there would be a knock on the door and someone would ask if I could talk to them or their daughter/son, friend who had been diagnosed with Epilepsy. I was honoured to be asked and a lot of these people were distraught. I made them a cup of tea and tried to tell them that their life was not over; it's not the end of the world. You can live a fairly normal life. Also I explained that we are all different, you have to 'listen' to your body. When you are tired, don't push yourself too much. (Famous last words for me!). I hope I helped. I can tell when my sugar level drops, I wee 'sugar puffs' (it smells like them) and I go very cold. Usually I have a cup of sweet tea and then eat a banana or a bar of chocolate and I begin to feel more 'normal'. It works for me (comes in useful when in the middle of town!)

Anyway we had a family pow wow and the kids thought it was a great idea for us to foster and if there were any problems we would face them when they arose.

Andy & I were both at home to give these children the love and care that they needed.

It is a very strict interview, understandably and we got through the first stage, eight more to go! Social workers came to see us and they were happy. We had our own social worker who communicated with us and we got right to the last stage, then there was a knock on the door. She stood there with tears running down her face. I invited her in and knew the answer. They had turned us down because of me being an epileptic and I might drop the baby. What Baby! We had asked for older children?! I broke down, I didn't want to face the world and shut myself away for days. Kirsti and Ross got me out of it and I saw how lucky I was and I wasn't meant to be a foster mother, so what could I be?

I went on a job hunt and was turned down at every one for the same reason, I am an Epileptic, and they didn't see me as a capable person but what they read in textbooks.

In 1989 our solicitor who had been working to get compensation for Andy's accident said we were 'close' and we were entitled to an interim payment. We thought great, pay some bills off! Also treat the kids. They had both suffered, but hardly moaned. Ross was upset the most as he had lost his Dad who used to run around with him and play football with him. It took us all a long time to come to terms with Andy being a different person almost, but he gradually began to accept being disabled. This payment helped and we started to feel hope and that it wouldn't be long before Andy received his compensation.

After much discussion and sleepless nights we decided to open a joke shop for the children in the village and maybe Andy could do portraits, so I went to our local Job centre which was then in Heanor to ask if they would help with this. The man there just took one look at me and asked if I was mad. He said why did I want to do this when I was getting disability? Pride was the reason. There was no help from them then. It made me even more determined to earn my own living and not scrounge off the Government!

So armed with a business plan I went to the bank to try and get a business loan. I was successful and with it we had a small extension built around the back of the house for the darkroom and a very small shop. Also we bought a new shed which housed the jokes and novelties. We used some of the loan to send the children to a PGL camp, which they loved and they really deserved. Andy would work for me therapeutically, which meant he could work a few hours a week and still get disability. I went off disability and in the summer of 1990 opened Bygone Photo's and Crafts.

Customers would come down the drive and around the back. The Joke Shed worked very well except when it was raining! There was lots of room and shelf space. Luckily it was alarmed because that winter when it was snowing, somebody tried to break in and as soon as they got their sticky little fingers through the walls of the shed, the infra red sensor picked them up and started the alarm off which is very loud! By the time we got outside all we could see was blood in the snow. We spent that week going around the local pubs to look at people's hands!

I dressed up smartly and went around door knocking to persuade people to have a portrait and tell them about the joke shop. This is how I got our first portrait sitter. Our sitting room doubled as a photographic studio. It also meant that I had to keep it tidy all the while! From humble beginnings…………………..

After about a month a 6 foot 2 inch man asked if I would make him a Fairy costume. He worked with disabled children and I had already made him a waterproof coat a few years earlier. I had a sewing machine and was always sewing something.

I was terrified, but he had confidence in me, so I made him it and he was over the moon with his Fairy outfit. This became lovingly known as the Fat Fairy and with me being large (about 16 stones by now as I took more tablets a day to cope with running a business) it wasn't discriminatory.

That was my very first costume and I ended up with over 700 of them, most of them hand made by me. By October 1990, I had made 25 costumes and hung them on a rail in our bedroom downstairs. This was our first changing room and the customers would come in and sit on the bed! A lot of these remained loyal to me and it was through them that I got more customers. Word and mouth recommendation works around here and I thank them all xx.

I remade these early outfits and we decided to go the whole hog as a Fancy dress shop.

I owned and ran a Fancy Dress Business for 16 years and loved every minute of it, well nearly………….

This was a new Beginning and we had a lot to learn.

I looked around what Fancy Dress shops had to offer and found our nearest one was in Swanwick, owned by Kate. So I took a deep breath and phoned her up and asked her if she objected to me opening a Fancy Dress shop in Underwood. She was a great help and a friend since then.

I noticed that the costumes in most of the Fancy Dress shops only went up to a size 14 and seeing as I was a size 18/20 by then I thought that this was very unfair. Not all of us are this size by eating too much! So I made lots of large costumes and this became my saviour. I sewed for hours, sometimes through the night, just to get a good range of costumes. There was and always will be another one I would like to make.

In 1993 after 3 years of struggling with a hefty business loan and often not being able to take a wage, Andy received his compensation money. It had taken 7 years. We decided to rebuild again! Another storey was added for our son's bedroom, so we could move our bedroom upstairs with an en-suite. This left the room downstairs to become the new shop. With another storey at the back and a large insulated Garage for a studio and storage, it looked brilliant!

After working in a very pokey shop we now had a 'proper' one, it was still small but big enough for us. With the shop being at the side of the house if I had a bad day, I could just about cope. I would collapse on the settee in between customers and Andy would help.

He didn't have too many portraits which suited him as he still was having problems with his leg, so he was there for me and I was there for him.

The only downer was losing on of our gardens as the stipulation was we had to have a customer car park. The Garage was used mainly in November and December for portraits but we had some great parties in there. Still do!

So, that Fairy costume started me off in the Fancy dress business and gave me the confidence to make some more. Thank you Steve for asking me to make that Fairy.

6 Penny the Clown

WHEN I FIRST STARTED the business in 1990 I quickly realised that I needed to go out and advertise more. I had already gone around the village door knocking and had success with that.

One of my friends suggested that I did a local car boot to sell some of the jokes and novelties. So I designed and photocopied some flyers and that Sunday stood at a car boot.

This went quite well for a couple of weeks, I never took a lot of money, but thought the rent was worth paying for because of all the advertising I did whilst there. Selling the Jokes and Novelties was a bonus. As I wasn't allowed to drive, a friend would take me and drop me off at the car boot. Also Andy wasn't keen on me going on my own so Kirsti, my daughter (now nearly 13yrs) used to come and help, but she became pretty bored.

We had face paints for sale and someone asked if we face painted. 'No' I replied, 'Not this week, but we will do next week!' Panic stations, I hadn't face painted in years! So all that next week Kirsti and I practised face painting on each other. The next Sunday we started face painting.

Whilst we were doing this someone spotted us and asked if we would face paint at their fete and as I did fancy dress, would I come dressed up? 'Of course' I replied, 'No problem!' Panic stations again, what the hell would I wear? Kirsti said she would let me do the face painting which was very magnanimous of her, but she suggested that I dressed as a clown. This was a great idea as I am a large woman and a baggy clown top would be comfortable to wear. So I made one and finished it off with a bright pair of leggings, stripy socks a pink or blue wig and a pair of old boots with painted spots on. Penny the Clown was born!

As I dressed as a clown I tried to juggle in between customers. So I stood there thinking that I was getting the hang of it when a man walked by and shouted; 'You've dropped your balls love, you're not a very good clown are you!' That made me practise more.

I was a bag of nerves, but I became Penny the Clown and I loved face painting. Soon I was asked to do Children's parties but I had to tell them I was an epileptic, also I needed collecting and returning home. Some of them said; 'No problem' and they hired me, some just hung up and some said that they would get back to me but didn't. I had to charge less because of my disability. Ho Hum, such is life!

That first Winter I started doing Copperfield Fairs indoor car boots in Selston. These were and are run by Kathryn and Richard who are great people and good friends. They helped me when no one else would. Thank you to them both.

It was their suggestion to get a taxi to the car boots as it was only in the next village and this worked very well until the taxi driver started complaining. I couldn't have carried on if it wasn't for my Dad, a wonderful caring man, who said he would take and collect me from all car boots and fetes etc. So now I was working most Sundays as Penny the clown and in the summer also doing at least 9 Gala's and fetes. This was hard work and I used to come home shattered, I couldn't move. I was living on sweet coffee and luck. I was always tired and my back started playing up with all the bending over to face paint. Andy was doing most of the housework and cooking, but he didn't mind.

We were closed on Mondays so at least that was a rest day, of sorts.

At first when working outdoors I used a paste table, and then we bought an old stall, and then added a closed trailer to this which stood at the back of the stall.

By this time I employed Saturday assistants in the shop and they used to come out with me and Kirsti. Emma and Kirsti really got on, but they both used to hate the cold and there was many a time I realised that they had both disappeared. I heard laughter and they were both hiding in the trailer out of the cold and wind!

In 1993 we decided to buy a small caravan. We painted on this bright blue clouds, balloons and a clown. It proved to be a Godsend! We had a curtained off Porta Loo area, a cooker and bright comfy seats. When we worked 'out' we now took more stock; jokes and novelties which grew as the shop expanded. The van replaced the trailer and became known as the Clown van. It was invaluable especially if it rained as I could face paint inside it. At least we had somewhere to shelter. I learnt to dash to the loo in two minutes flat in between my little customers!

On Sundays it was a family affair and Andy would come with us to help set up. He also cooked egg and bacon butties and copious cups of coffee.

Kirsti helped until her children were born; twin boys March 1996.

It was hard work but good fun. Not so good when we didn't take a lot of money though but we always had a laugh.

My left arm was always browner than my right as I used to place my left hand on top of the child's head to keep it still as I painted their face. Mind you, one summer we did the galas etc in our wellies as it rained so much. It was surprising and heart warming to see how many people turned up despite the weather.

I've even met Kathy Staff at Bakewell Gala, but I was so Gobsmacked that I just stared and smiled at her like an idiot!

After a while we got busier in the shop on Fridays and Saturdays. Tuesdays were nicknamed smelly day as this was when we got the dirty fancy dress back in to wash.

I also found myself turning down more and more children's parties and then cutting down on Galas and fetes. This was upsetting as I enjoyed doing them, but they were tiring. The one

I really missed was the Christmas fair at Selston which was really festive! Even when I cut these out I still worked too many hours, my health and my family were suffering. I needed to slow down to enjoy my life and my grandchildren.

I still love face painting though now I suffer with arthritis and it is harder to do.

People still know me as Penny the clown.

7 *Regressing to the Joke Shed*

I KNOW IT SOUNDS weird having a garden shed for a joke
shop, but it worked really well. The shed was new and we
reinforced the inside by screwing wooden panels to the walls
and after the attempted break in added wire mesh to the window.
It was fully alarmed and the door was fitted with several locks. It
had lots of shelves and even a light!

There was room for me and at least two customers; I must
admit I was thinner then!

Our first Jokes & Novelties order was about £2,000, which
bought a lot of stock in 1990.

We spent ALL day unpacking it and playing with the stock in
our bedroom which was quite large. We sat on the bed surrounded
by all these amazing things!

Ross and Kirsti helped us and we will never forget that first
order, especially Ross. He held up a can of fart spray and
whooped; 'Cool, fart spray!' I took the lid off and sprayed him
with it-BIG MISTAKE! This stuff is foul. We had to strip the bed
and Ross went in the shower with all his clothes on. We had to
vacate the room. Evil Stinky stuff, it took hours to get the stench
out of our room even with the windows open.

I learned a lesson that day, do not spray it indoors!

I only sold the spray occasionally and after receiving
complaints from a lot of locals I stopped selling it altogether.

When we first started up, nobody locally was selling what we
were. We were different and like a breath of fresh air (a customers
words, not mine) and the masks were/are amazing. It was a lot
easier to sell things before the supermarkets muscled in and
started getting greedy.

Ross helped unpack the stock. It was delivered in large
washing machine size boxes, so I welcomed all the help I could

get, it was long hard work and all he wanted in payment was stock. No problem, he was a great help.

As we acquired more customers we naturally sold more and more stock and I soon discovered that there was a niche in the market for this. I branched out on wigs; make up, accessories such as hats and dressing up kits.

We even sold Wellingtons in the summer months as nobody locally sold them until Jonathon James started up. I did quite well with them!

My mark up was lower than the large shops I didn't make 200% plus, like they did and I sold stock quite quickly, which was better than having them sitting on a shelf.

Over the years the Fancy dress business has improved and changed so much that you can now buy a ready made costume at a good price. This wasn't so when I started and each year I had to make my costumes and stock look better.

I outgrew the shed and was glad when we moved in our 'proper' shop with a front shop door.

It even got harder selling jokes & novelties on the car boots, but at least I was one of the first to do it!

I soon learned that we had to open late some evenings for those who couldn't come in the day time and I started doing evening appointments, which was really tiring, but necessary.

I will always remember opening day when my Uncle Peter, who was a Deacon, came to see me and he bought a Whoopee cushion. He said I was very enterprising which I took as a great compliment. He was a great man and I will never forget him for coming out of his way to support me when I needed it the most.

From little acorns…………………………….

8 Sizes, Smells & Washing

I LEARNT A LOT and met a lot of people whilst I was running the shop and it was an experience that I will never forget. One thing I had to learn was to keep quiet! (Difficult for me) Also I didn't tell customers what I was, some guessed when I nearly passed out on them, but this wasn't very often.

One of the things that used to make me laugh was the amount of women who wouldn't own up to what size they really were. Some of them lived in a sort of fairy land and went around pretending that they were a size 14 when in reality they were a size 20!

A size 26 female walked into the shop one day and what did she want to be? Laura Croft! Did she really think that she would get away with looking like Angelina Jolie? If she has looked a little bit like her heroine it would have helped and after biting my tongue (which could do without extra biting on!) and swallowing the sarcasm, I was polite and tried to sway her away from making a complete fool of her self. I suggested a pair of shorts and a top, not too tight, then buying some toy guns to strap to her thighs and a wig to complete the picture. She was very happy with that and you I wasn't being cruel here, but this woman had a lot of 'wobbly bits' and she was hoping to attract a boyfriend. All I tried to teach her was that sometimes less is not best! I mean I am large and I love dressing up, but even I couldn't get away with dressing up say as Julia Roberts, maybe Dawn French, but even she is younger and better looking than me!

It was amazing when a woman used to tell me that she was a size 12 and then when she couldn't get into a costume would remark; 'This is a small 12!' I would look at them and say; 'No, I always make them a bit larger if anything, but I am a size 20 cough, cough, and I've lots of costume that fit me so there we will easily find something for you as you are a lot smaller than me'

That usually put them at their ease and then they would truthfully tell me what size they were which made it easier for me to do my job. I didn't care that they were bigger than a 12, I only wanted to find a costume that would fit them properly and that they felt good in.

A happy customer would usually come back and bring someone else.

I had a lot of really good looking women come in the shop with great figures, but they didn't think so. It was hard work telling them otherwise. This was completely different from the big headed ones who swanned in reeking of expensive perfume which made me sneeze and they thought they looked gorgeous in everything.

Malodorous customers were awful! Most of the time there were unaware of this personal problem. Sometimes a whole family would come in and the smell of BO would arrive in the shop before them! I just hate that smell. I am quite fussy……..

If someone followed them in and their nose went up, I said 'Sorry, we have just had a guy in with smelly feet!' and then I would spray the room with lavender spray.

If it was the summer then I could open the door, but sometimes even that didn't help.

The trouble was a customer following them in might think the smell was from my costumes and not them!

The other problem was them trying costumes on and when they picked one that took a lot of washing I would say; 'Sorry but that one is not available'. Hopefully they would only try on a few costumes, as I would have to wash all of them that they didn't hire, later on that night. If you left one smelly costume upstairs then the whole lot would stink.

You had to move them quickly and discretely downstairs into the sitting room. One of my best excuses was; 'Is this the top/dress that needs sewing?' and raise my eyebrows at one of 'my girls'. They usually caught on and took it down stairs.

This was a good excuse when I didn't feel too good and I would leave the customer to my staff. A cup of sweet tea and then I could hopefully finish the hire.

The worst smell in the changing room was smelly feet. Many a time I have turned my back and said; 'Sorry I won't be a moment, my hay fever is playing me up!' I would sit on the stairs, take a big gulp on air and then go back trying not to breathe too deeply.

Luckily most of my customer smelt lovely and didn't moan too much

One of the most asked questions was; 'Do you wash all your costumes?' I wanted to reply; 'Of course not, I hire them out smelly!' I was neurotic about the costumes being clean and I even used to do the 'sniff test' after each outfit was tried on, which was an awful job. I always used to thank the customers for smelling clean.

I often got asked if we had an old woman in the back doing the laundry. Yes, me! People thought we sent the whole lot to the dry cleaners, which would have cost a fortune. I had a bad experience with them once when I sent a 50 year old Teddy Boy suit to be cleaned. It came back with the colours faded and still smelt.

When making costumes I sometimes used drip dry material or hand wash material. I didn't like using nylon which made a rod for my own back and I had to iron a lot of the Fancy Dress. Our own clothes hardly ever got ironed! All the accessories were hand washed on the kitchen table. The costumes were washed in the washing machine (we had two) or hand washed. If it was a nice day then I hung them outside for a blow, and then hung around our sitting room on two long poles fastened to the ceiling.

Honestly sometimes it was like sitting in a clearing in a dark wood!

Everything was ironed or if it was an 'animal' brushed. Even the wigs were shampooed and conditioned, then hung to drip dry over the bath. We then hung them around our large fire in the sitting room to dry and then we brushed them.

Andy was an expert wig washer and brusher!

Enough of my ramblings of one of my pet hates of the job…washing!

We also used to use our sitting room as a spare changing room when we were really busy and for large groups. There was a full length mirror in there and we tried to keep the room reasonably tidy which was a losing battle some of the time. My husband's idea of tidy and my idea of tidy are different! Using the sitting room made us more work as we had to carry the costumes up and down the stairs; most of them got left on the ceiling rails and we ended up putting them away late at night.

Some customers were quite rude when they walked into the sitting room. One looked around and said; 'Do you live here!' I felt like replying; 'No the large TV is just for show', but just pretended not to hear them. Some were even ruder and said; 'God how do you live like this! Charming, cheeky sods, it felt like I lived in a hovel! This really used to upset me as we had put ourselves out to make their time shorter with us and they were rude about my home. I am quite sensitive and this didn't help with my self confidence.

One woman called our home bohemian. I didn't know what it meant so I just sorted her out as quickly as possible. Afterwards I found out that she was on about our knick knacks, I mean if someone had bought you some thing, you have to display it, don't you?

During the busy seasons; October to December a lot of customers used to say; 'I bet you make a bomb here!' Well, after taking a few steps back I replied; 'If you call £5,000 a year making a bomb then yeah I'm loaded! If they kept going on about it and why I kept running the shop I would just look at them and say; ' Look, I am an epileptic, this is my business and nobody can take it off me, it's mine and I love it' Usually they looked startled and didn't know what to say, but after that they treated me differently. Some of them accepted it, but others didn't come back to the shop again.

Maybe if I had known that I was going to run a laundry and I was always at everybody's beck and call then maybe, just maybe I might have done things differently.

Our shop was packed full of stock and when customers came in it was a squeeze. People would come in and say; 'Why don't you get a bigger shop? Well, we did think about it in 1996 when a large corner shop came up for rent in Eastwood, our nearest town. It would have been ideal; there was plenty of room for the costumes and more, plus car parking.

The trouble was that I would have had to bring the washing home and do it at night then take it back the next morning. There wasn't room there for it to dry. As I am not allowed to drive, it meant catching a bus or walking the 3 miles there every day. Also I would have had to employ more staff. With all the extra costs the hire of the costumes would have had to rise.

The main disadvantage was that if I had a bad day I couldn't rest up on the settee in between customers. So all in all was this a good thing? I decided; No and to keep the business small.

The thing was the more customers I got the more work it was for me, so I was working longer hours and missing out on my family.

 Just keep smiling is my motto!

9 Making Costumes, Where & How?

I could write a whole book on why and how I made the costumes and so that I don't bore the pants off you, I will pick just a few.
I love watching films, so a lot of my ideas came from these, plus I love people watching.

Whether we were out for the day, shopping or on holiday, something would catch my eye. For instance in the early nineties we started going on coach holidays (our one way of touring around the country) in January or February as they were reasonably priced and this is when I got my New Year wages. We were staying in Exmouth and we had a 'walk' (me pushing Andy in a wheelchair) near the docks and we spotted a shop called; 'Who threw that?' It was full of amazing clothes! We ended up going into our personal overdraft, (this was a recurring thing over the years) and bought an American Highway patrol gun belt. This was put together with a lovely fringed suede mans jacket and some other items which I already had and it became The Texan ranger; Burt Reynolds. This was how a lot of costumes came together, when I already had some 'bits' and it just needed the right one to complete it. I bought loads of things from that shop, but the gun belt has always stayed in my mind as it was unusual.

Every year I would write a list of costumes that I would like to make, but more often then not a customer would walk into the shop and ask; 'Would you like to buy this?' That was how I acquired my American Officer. It was a beautiful suit and one of my favourites and I was very tempted not to auction it off. An American was visiting relatives in England and had brought it with him. He wanted £200 in the beginning and I couldn't afford it, so he went around all the other shops with it. He came back to me with a revised offer which left me skint, but it was worth it, I have seen mothers weep when they saw their sons in that suit!

Every year a town near us called Kimberley ran the Pram race and regular groups would hire off me for their themed 'pram'. One group, most of who worked at the Leisure centre came in and asked me for Humpty Dumpty. I didn't have one, but they got around me and that is how Humpty was born. Not a costume for people with weak bladders as once you were in it that was it! I made quite a few costumes for the runners of the Pram race and they were great people to sew for and a good laugh. I can remember the last one as they dressed as Star Wars and I made Chewbacca for them. I was really proud of Chewy!

Early on in the business I decided that I wasn't making enough costumes for the demand I was getting, so in 1993 I went to an Auction of Derby Playhouse costumes. It was held in the cattle market showroom and it was freezing! I had ringed quite a few of the outfits that I wanted but they went for to much money. I ended up with some good outfits.

One of the best was a panto Dame. It had a huge sticky out skirt which had plaster hearts hanging off it. Now this skirt wouldn't fit in the washing machine so I had to wash it over the bath! It finished off drying hanging from the beams in the sitting room and then I had to repaint the little hearts.

We often went to Scotland as we love it there and we usually went on a coach tour which enabled us to enjoy the countryside.

So all my Scotsmen came from ..Scotland! Every time we went up there we came back with something like children's bagpipes, (much cheaper than adults) also tartan material and kilts (ladies as they are cheaper and I remade them to fit men). When I made Braveheart, I went into a Tartan shop and asked if they had that type of tartan. The assistant laughed and told me it was a Hollywood one! So I chose a similar one which was washable and a stretchy material. I designed a kilt with pleats that were top stitched down and an elasticised waist. The suede jerkin was made out of my old suede skirt which I made holes in to thread 'stitches' through. This was another of my favourites and very popular with the customers. Andy was brilliant at making sword scabbards out of cardboard covered in leather left over bits and glue. We got through tons of glue.

When I was making a costume I was calm and lost myself in them. The cutting out is the most stressful bit!

Italy is the leather capital of the world, so to speak, so when we discovered a holiday coach firm that took you to a camp site in Italy, left you there for a week or so and then took you home, we fell in love with the country. I closed the shop for a couple of weeks in September and it was great unwinding in a warm country where people are lovely and you can do what you want when you want. Also we bought cowboy belts there as they were half the price than at home. I would love visiting the markets wherever we were and always came home with loads of beautiful and unusual ribbons and buttons. These were incorporated them into whatever costume I was making at that moment.

I loved making capes and they covered a multitude of sins! I had some gorgeous black velour material and made these into capes with sequins on for the witches.

On a coach trip to Canada (our 25th Wedding anniversary) we bought a proper Mountie Hat, cowboy shirts and other items. I parcelled them up and sent them home. That Hat looked so good, in fact I put off making the outfit for ages as I was worried that I couldn't. Then I thought; 'How does anyone in England know what a Mountie looks like?' I did my best and was pleased with the result. It was always a head turner. Andy was really upset that we put it in the Auction. Anyway it's a good excuse to go back to Canada to buy a new hat!

During the same trip we went to San Francisco and visited a Fancy Dress shop which was absolutely amazing! It was jam packed full of stuff. I bought a PVC Wonder Woman Suit which the owner thought was for me and she suggested a bigger size! When I explained she wanted to know all about fancy dress shops in England.

That outfit wasn't cheap, but that was typical of me as I always wanted the costumes to look good and like their originals.

There aren't many super hero women about and that is why I ended up making three Xena outfits. All in different sizes, the largest was a size 20/22. They were very popular and made out of PVC, leather lots of studs and buttons, most of them hand sewn. They took ages to make but were worth it as most women like to 'kick butt' every so often!

Andy & I love Sci-if and I designed the Star wars and Trek uniforms as soon as possible. I bought the masks from America and this was way before online shopping, so they cost about £50 each, plus postage. I ordered Dart Vade, Dart Maul, Yoda and they took over 8 weeks to arrive! Andy loved the Dart Vade one.

The other hire masks; the Flintstones's, Batman's, Catwoman, Star Trek Spock and the Space Hero were bought from the Mask Shack in Leicestershire. They were brilliant and really made the costumes.

The hire capes were double with an inner and an outer and for Batman I used a material which looked leathery. Dart Vade had three layers plus the chest so it was a heavy outfit and you couldn't wear it if you were claustrophobic. One man who hired it was so tired that when he went out he sat down at the party and fell asleep, but nobody noticed! He woke up after an hour and thoroughly enjoyed himself.

Andy and Kirsti stood over me when I made the Star Trek outfits as they wanted them to look like the real thing! It was nerve racking! I must have done a good job as Andy asked me to make him one just like it, which he still has.

I used to watch films and then pause them over and over again to get a costume right which used to drive Andy nuts! I did this with Snow White and the seven dwarfs, the 3 Musketeers which were a mixture of the Oliver Reed film and The man in the Iron Mask. These took ages to make as there were 3 of them and I was really proud of them. Andy looked great as a musketeer.

My first two person animal was Daisy the cow and she had a wonderful personality! My friend Pauline and I did the 3 mile Underwood run in this, but she was faster then me and we soon split up. Daisy velcroed up in the middle. So there was me miles behind wandering along wearing the back bit with the cow's udders! It was good fun though! The udders had to be sewn back on every time it went out. She was so popular that I ended up remaking Daisy three times.

I think that in all my creations there was a bit of me in them.

Felley Players an Underwood Drama group used to hire costumes off me and for one Panto they hired Daisy. Nicky and Rachel were in Daisy and they were very funny. I was very proud to see my costumes and they all looked good in them. Marine who is a good friend of mine just brought these people to life; there is a lot of talent there.

Unfortunately I didn't go to watch as many of the plays and panto's as I would have liked as I was always working. I thank them and all the other groups from hiring off me.

One of the downsides to creating costumes was that mine and Andy's wardrobes got raided quite regularly, especially for shirts. I did buy some things from second hand shops, but not many.

For patterns, a bought a few and I made some and some costumes I just cut out. I just got a feeling and followed it. The carrot was one of these and it was like a long orange sleeping bag!

I remade some outfits a few times. The Mask was one of these and I remade it twice, bought 3 new shirts and loads of ties because the customers kept losing them.

I just like making things.

10   *Work is Not Everything*

I WAS ALWAYS TIRED, even when I started opening at 10am and not 9am (as I used to) in the mornings as not many people came in before 10am. Also I worked some nights when I had evening appointments with customers. At first we opened on Tuesdays to Saturdays plus on a lot of Sundays doing Galas, Fetes and car boots. I was young in my 30's in the beginning, but over the years my health suffered. I started having more fits. This was due to lack of sleep. My joints started giving me jip, mainly due to all the falls and breaks and sprains that I have suffered over the years. I started taking more vitamin tablets. I had problems with my stomach, due to all the epilepsy tablets that I had taken and I found it hard digesting food. I have to keep clear of preservatives and saccharin. I started taking kelp tablets every day to help my tummy. The one thing that has suffered is my tongue and gums, which are now quite sensitive. As soon as my tongue heals I bite it again even when I am having a petit, Sometimes I have these whilst I'm asleep as things go over and over in my brain and then I wake up with blood on the pillow and a sore mouth. Bonjela helps and Daktarin. I get used to waiting for drinks and food to cool before I eat/drink it or else I would burn my mouth. Ice cream is too cold and I have to wait until it's 'warmer' or nearly melted!

I look 'normal', people don't realise how much a struggle some days are and you have to put a brave face on. I have to push myself. By this time we had discovered Acupuncture for Andy which helped with his pain and once a month he was able to walk more, but it wasn't cheap and not on the NHS then. I went with him sometimes when I couldn't stand the pain in my joints any more and it eased them but not for long. A friend introduced me to aromatherapy oils which Andy rubbed onto my back and joints and this helped. When it got too bad Nurofen was our best friend!

This is how we got through running the village Gala, which we started in 2000, that day is brilliant but exhausting! I also went for physiotherapy at the hospital and that helped with my back but after a few sessions they said they couldn't do any more for me. Then I went to a specialist about my knees as they had been through hell and were always swollen. She took one look at the x rays, then at me and said; 'We can't do anything for you as this has been self afflicted'. Pardon?!? Are you real, do you think I have sat there hitting them with a hammer? We were struck dumb and just walked out disgusted!

I had to see the doctor at least every 6 months or else he would phone me to go and see him.

He asked if I went anywhere on my own as this was unadvisable. It was a sort of unwritten thing between me and Andy that I had someone with me most of the time. I couldn't even go swimming on my own, but I didn't have time to go anyway with all the work. The Doctor said that I had to start seeing the specialist again as I should not be having the amount of fits that I was having. So I started seeing the specialist once every 3 months again. Basically he told me to cut down on my hours or finish the shop. There wasn't a lot of help for epileptics then or support groups, you just got on with living the best way that you could.

So I took a long look at the business and after 13 years of working long hours I cut them down. I decided that from February to September I would do a 4 day week; Tuesday, Thursday, Friday and Saturday.

I cut all car boots and Galas out except one; Brinsley. This was our next village and I loved doing that one. This helped, but what people didn't realize that when the shop was closed I didn't stop working. I 'caught up' at night and when I didn't have any customers in the shop it was bliss to sew a costume with no interruptions. I also sat and sewed the endless repairs and the hand sewing on the new costumes. I did these whilst I watched the television so at least I was sitting down and I didn't mind doing this as I wanted them to look their best.

I loved having Mondays off, it was 'our' day (well most of it) and we tried not to do any washing, sewing or ironing on that day. I had to do the shopping in the morning and usually went with my Dad & Josie, but afterwards the day was ours. I looked forward to Mondays as we could go for a 'walk' (Andy in his electric wheel chair and me walking, which cut down on the places we could go, but at least we got out in the summer months). Sometimes I was too tired to do anything. On the other days the washing carried on being done after closing time and the mounds of ironing.

As well as this, customers who couldn't make it during opening times used to come to the house door to return costumes. Or they just turned up at any time of the day just to see if 'I could help them'. In other words, I can't be bothered to visit you in opening hours so open up now and serve me! Sometimes the considerate customers used to telephone before hand and make an appointment, no problem. We had more evening customers from October to December .

Our personal washing, ironing and cleaning of the house got done when there wasn't a lot of fancy dress to launder. So usually our laundry was done on Sundays or at midnight on any night that the washers were free. I ended up ironing our clothes in the morning when we needed them, so our ironing pile was always as big as a mountain.

I loved the job and most of my customers, but mostly making the costumes.

11 Seasons

THE FANCY DRESS BUSINESS, like a lot of other businesses, work around the seasons.

As I said before, we built the shop onto the side of the house, so the sitting room is adjacent to it. There is a large bay window in the sitting room and we used this as a display window, so from the front it looked like one large shop!

The bay window is large and quite deep as it covers nearly one wall. I used to hang a net curtain across the back of it which would give us a bit of privacy as quite a few children would sit on the wall outside it. They would often tap on the window and sometimes when they did this I would poke my head under the net curtain and pull a face at them which made them jump!

When we first opened I changed the window every month, but this became less as we got busier. We lit the street up at Christmas time with this window and the small shop window blazing away! No wonder the electricity bill was so high. I tried to alter the window every Christmas when I would buy something new from the warehouse. We had moving singing snowman, dancing Santa's, a sleigh with reindeer, changing light Christmas trees and lots more.

The children would look in the window as they passed it on their way to and from school and I loved watching their faces break into smiles. There was one little boy who looked every morning and he loved it when I changed the window. You could hear him shouting; 'Mummy look they've changed it and it's really cool!' That made my day.

I put seasonal stock in the window, such as fairy wings and crowns for Christmas and I would spend ages looking for something, before I realised it was in the window!

Each year I ordered more stock in and the problem was that I never knew how much to order and my stock bill was always huge each September to December. I had to use Andy's overdraft in September and I would pay him back, which was always a big worry.

After the New Year we quickly changed the Christmas window and there usually wasn't any stock left, so it didn't take long. Funnily enough the Christmas after we closed I got the 'toys' out as I missed the window dressed up and it looked great!

The January window was very simple as we were very tired by then. We didn't have the energy to do a lot. It was a few poly heads with wigs or hats on and that sort of thing.

My way of getting through the Christmas and New Year mayhem was sleeping. I used to sit on the settee and just drop off!

The next theme window was Valentines Day; 14th February, which was an easy window to do. Basically I went around the shop grabbing all the red things that I could see, such as boas, wigs, and hats etc. I cut hearts out of red card and used red material and cloths. Whatever I put in the window usually helped to sell stock which was good as it was a bit lean for takings until spring when it usually picked up a bit.

Then there was spring. I had fun with spring and we used all sorts for the window. We had a bunny window, a daffodil window, a duck window, a green and yellow window, in fact anything that made it look happy and bright.

Good job I collected soft toys as they came in useful.

Adult costumes were too big to fit in the window so we sometimes used children's. One year we took ages stuffing the children's rabbit and as soon as it was put in the window it was hired out! We used plastic carrier bags for stuffing as they clean and it was recycling. They were even good for putting in masks when we ran out of poly heads!

One summer we filled the base of the window with sand and buckets and spades. It was messy but the children loved it. I was forever cleaning sand off the carpet!

There was always a theme to do; Pudsey bear, Red Nose day etc.

Halloween was one of my favourites and one year we made a large cardboard coffin with an inflatable skeleton in it. It filled the window! There's always gory stuff for sale at this time of the year and these went in the window. We used to put a large branch in there to hang things on and used lots of false cobweb wool. (Great stuff and I still put it around the back door at Halloween, but it's a sod to get off the rose bushes as it sticks to the thorns!) Add a low light and the Halloween window is born.

The worst change over and the most welcome was from Halloween to the Christmas window as it had to be done very quickly and there always lots of things to put away. I usually ended up doing this late at night and it was lovely to have a bright happy window.

The season windows marked the differences in the 'buying' months in the shop. As I have already said the busiest ones were October to December when I was open for 6 days a week plus evening customers. Then January and February were mostly washing and ironing. Also we tried to get away then to recharge our batteries. People still came into the shop to hire costumes in these months as every day is someone's birthday, anniversary, hen night and stag night.

Spring brought people in to dress as bunnies, chicks and eggs (humpty). Summer brought in people to dress up at Gala's, fete's or summer fairs. So there was usually a celebration going off somewhere. Sometimes people just fancied a party, good on 'em, have fun!

I had a lot of customers who fell in love with a costume and used to keep coming back and hiring the same one. I thought this was a bit bonkers as they had the pick from hundreds, people are very funny!

My life was stressful and tiring, but never boring. I loved the fact that I never knew who was going to walk through that door.

12   *Things Left in and on Costumes*

IT'S AMAZING what people leave behind in pockets of outfits and in the fancy dress bags. (I used to fold the outfit and accessories in a new black bin bag to make it easier to carry).

The worst one was in the early days when I plunged my hand into the returned bag to check the outfit and it came out covered in poo!!! I ran to the loo and promptly threw up. The customer's dirty bitch of a friend had had an accident and left her dirty undies in the bag. Needless to say she lost her deposit and I lost a customer, which I wasn't that worried about. This taught me a good lesson, first of all; tip the contents out and don't put your hand into the bag.

The best one was when I was checking through the pockets of a returned cowboy costume and I found a purse with £50 in it! I bet you're thinking; 'It must be your lucky day!' Well, I thought that for two seconds and then telephoned the customer who was a regular and who owned the local garden centre. They are a great couple and always hired a Santa and elves from me every Christmas, plus outfits for parties. She was so pleased, that when she came to collect her purse she brought me a large box of chocolates as a thank you......the way to a woman's heart. (Especially me as I am a chocoholic) No wonder I keep putting weight on! I could have kept the £50, but it would have plagued me for ever.

Even when someone used to leave small change in the pockets I would phone them up. If they never came for it then I put it in the charity box, until somebody pinched it!

I learned in my early years that it was best to be honest and it has always proved to be right.

We had loads of lipsticks left behind, most of them grotty so I threw them away. There was a few cameras, tons of hankies, condoms new and used, socks (some really smelly!), watches, perfumes, nail varnishes and other weird things. I always felt sorry for the young men when I found a new packet of condoms in the pockets after News Years Eve. It meant that they hadn't had a lucky night! On one of these occasions I knew the young man who hired the costume, so thinking that he might need them, (I mean they aren't cheap to buy are they?) I put them in an envelope and posted them through his front door. It wasn't until I got home that Andy said; 'Do you realize that he lives with his Dad and what if he opens the envelope thinking that it was for him?' Whoops.

New condoms weren't a problem. The worst thing was forgetting to look in the pockets before putting the outfit in the washer & the tumble dryer, then and finding a 'used' (now washed & dry) condom in the bottom of the dryer...yuck! Needless to say, when this happened the whole lot went back in the washing machine. I also put a piece of material soaked in lavender essence in the tumble dryer to cleanse it.

Sick is gross to find, but luckily there wasn't many cases of this, wine and mud, yes, but not sick. Thank goodness my stomach couldn't have taken it!

There have been lots of 'dried' substances on outfits that have looked a bit 'iffy', but I just put them in the washer on their own, sometimes twice and that did the trick. The worst one of these was when Superman came back. It looked ok and I washed and drip dried it but when I was ironing it I noticed that it needed sewing on the crotch, (yet again).

So I turned it inside out and there was a nice white crusty stain! I screamed and shouted; 'Mucky bu**er!' It went back in the washer then I scrubbed it and it went back in the washer again. I mean I've heard of wet dreams, but please, not in a superman costume in bed. What are you, some sort of perverted super hero weirdo?

From then on I gingerly checked men's crotches, so to speak!

Women were the worst for muddy trouser bottoms, especially the 70's outfits. They like the trousers long to touch the floor, but they didn't think twice about lifting them up when trawling through puddles and muddy fields, so I often had to make a new pair as I couldn't get them clean. This was the same with long dresses and skirts.

Over the years I have collected remedies for cleaning certain things off costumes and when it came down to it, elbow grease and scrubbing it with a nail brush and soap was the best thing. Andy used to do this as he could scrub harder than me, but he hated it and used to curse at the 'dirty pigs' whilst doing this thankless chore.

Dish washer tablets were great for shifting hard stains. It was really funny when someone used our bathroom and there was something soaking in the bath. They would come out and give us funny looks. Once we had the Dragon outfit soaking with its head leaning over the bath. It was made out of a hardened sort of material and rubber and was too large for the washing machine. Well, a customer went to use the loo and she came out screaming!

Talking about the Dragon, the story of how we acquired it was interesting. One day a couple walked into the shop and asked if we bought fancy dress. I asked what they had and they beckoned me outside to their Volkswagen. Now this couple were travellers, but had not always been so. Inside the van was a large box. The man undid it and asked if I had ever watched Rod Hull's Pink Windmill Show. I replied that I had and he said with glee; 'This is Croc!' I was amazed. He explained that he used to work backstage and he was given one of the crocs. The couple wanted to swap Croc for two hires from me and I agreed. They were going to a medieval wedding and this sounded very fair.

Because of copyright I called Croc a Dragon and made him wings and trousers. After repairing him he looked great and every so often he was hired out for a pagan/druid wedding. One man who hired it out for this said he had a great time, but the only trouble was that the dragon's tummy was so big that he had a problem getting on his motor bike! Also he had to take the head off as he couldn't see well enough to drive. I was amazed. He wanted to fly to the wedding and this was his idea of that!

The dragon took some cleaning, but our motto was; it's got to be clean enough for us to want to wear it.

As well as things left on and in costumes there were always bits of costumes left behind and Batman fell into this category. Their masks were specially made. Once when a Batman was returned the young man who hired it was very sheepish so I knew that something had happened to it. He said; 'Sorry Pen and I will pay for a new one, but somebody has pinched the mask' How, I asked? He looked at the floor and then went onto say that he was in a club and he had fancied this girl for ages and had actually got talking to her. He took the mask off and put it on the window sill to give her a kiss and that was the last he saw of it.

It turned out to be an expensive kiss as he paid me £25 (trade, how could I make a profit?) for a new mask.

He was a regular and this happened at New Year which was when most things went missing from costumes. Batman's leggings used to disappear quite often.

One apologetic young man said; 'Sorry about the leggings, but I was screwing my mate's wife and he came home unexpectedly and I had to leg it out of the window. I had time to grab the boots and pants but left the leggings behind!'

The mind boggles. Needless to say that time Batman went in the washer three times.

Smelly socks went straight in the bin, but one day after doing this, a customer came into the shop asking for her 'favourite' socks. So Andy had to quickly nip out the back and retrieve them from the bin! So from then onwards we kept them in a 'sock carrier back' for a few weeks (in the shed). If they weren't collected then they went in the bin.

When I closed the shop I had two drawers full of uncollected items.

The decent things such as cameras went to the Help the Aged Shop.

13   My Wonderful Assistants Who Kept Me Going!

AH, MY WONDERFUL GIRLS, without them I couldn't have kept going. They had a hard job with me as they had to read me, if you know what I mean and I expected a lot from them. They just didn't work for me they looked after me.

Kirsti, my daughter was the first and she worked for me, (as she put it), for love. Mind you when we were at Galas or fetes, she didn't do too badly out of me as she always went home with clothes or something! Kirsti has always been there to step in and give me a hand and after her twin boys were born this became more difficult, but she used to do a lot of ironing and I would buy her clothes in return. It was a good arrangement! She's not just my daughter but a good friend. Many a time she has picked me off the floor and washed me down, not a job a daughter should have to do to for her mum. Thank you.

Ross, my son helped when he could, but it really wasn't his thing. He would help me price up stock and do things behind the scenes so to speak. I couldn't have coped on the week that we closed the shop for good if he hadn't have been there.

The thing with Fancy dress is you either love it or you hate it and to work for me you had to live it! It had to be in your soul.

My next assistant was Amie who worked on Saturdays and when we went to Galas or fetes. She also worked Halloween week and Christmas and New Year. In fact after Amie left she would always pop in and see me and if we were busy, she would take her coat off and muck in and help! I was lucky with all my girls as they have all become good friends and keep in touch and help out. Amie was with me for quite a while and was a great asset to the business. She was capable of running the shop on her own, if I had sewing to do or had a bad day. I couldn't afford to pay her much as we weren't making a lot, but that didn't bother Amie.

My friend Samantha, who is a good laugh, used to help out when Kirsti couldn't and she came to Galas and fetes with me. The thing was not everyone wanted to give up their summer weekends to help me, but Sam loved helping so this worked well. Sam has a slim figure and she was one of my first models. The trouble was that I had to pad out the bigger costumes to fit her! She is very photogenic and loved doing the videos.

I can remember when we videoed her in Wonder Woman and as the original one had large boobs we had to use thick socks and make sure that they didn't whiz out when Sam twirled around! As Sam had a car she took me all over the place until she got a full time job and even then she helped out.

I was lucky to get such faithful assistants because sometimes when I told the Mums what I was I didn't see their daughters again. The ones who worked for me understood and saw me and not a person with a disability.

Next was Emma, the only one that I made cry which is something that I am not proud of! I didn't mean to but Emma was quite shy in the beginning and I am sometimes like a bear with a sore head. She soon settled in and realised that I am a bit of a softie underneath. I expected my assistants to work as hard as I did and you can't do that. It is hard training a new assistant in and there's a lot to learn about the shop and the way that I worked.

They have got to remember where all the costumes are and I had a sort of system.

There were also accessories and remembering what goes with what. Even I forgot this and would have to look in the fancy dress books to check if I had the right accessory. Some customers were quite picky and if the costume didn't look the same as the photograph or if they had different accessories they would complain!

The most important job was the booking in and out of the costumes. We had a hand written account of this so we knew where they were and we didn't double book. Then there was the stock and it was everywhere but it was an 'ordered chaos' as one customer put it. We all had to know where a certain item of stock was as it was embarrassing looking for it, not to mention the income that you could lose.

Then of course was the wonderful laundry! The shop had to look clean, 'tidyish' and well stocked. Emma took all this in her stride and worked hard. Her wages were peanuts, but she never complained. I used to give her and all the girls free stock as a make up for the wages. She worked well with the customers and was, still is a people person.

Emma is still a good friend and often comes to see us. She is now a Policewoman so her people skills have come in useful!

As well as Emma I had a young girl Keeley who would work for me on the days that Emma was unable to. She was very amenable and easy to get on with.

I am not sexist, but girls seem to work better in this business than boys. I am not that hard to work with, (I suppose I can be a bit fastidious!), but I often used to say; 'Have you got blu tack on your bum?' Which basically meant; Shift your butt and do some work? They soon learnt that I gave them good breaks and a lunchtime, but in between you worked. Even when we were really busy Andy and I made sure that the girls got a break. Nobody is superhuman!

I am afraid that I am from a generation that says; 'If you don't work for it then you'll never get it!

Also you never knew how busy it was going to be, some days it was really busy and others not so. When we got '10 minutes', I always used to say; 'Savour this moment and remember it in December and it will keep you going'. And it did.

After Emma left to train for the Police force I thought that I would never get an assistant as good as her and who was on the same wave length as me, but I was wrong.

Amie has two sisters and Charlotte was 14 years old. She asked if she could work for me on Saturdays and she took to it like a duck to water.

Charlotte has been a gem; she loved the business and enjoyed it. She was also very proud of the costumes which showed when she was trying to hire them out. I had a passion for the business because it was mine and I had built it up. I didn't expect the girls to share this but Charlotte did. She worked for me the longest and had a lot to put up with me in the last few years of opening as my health deteriorated and I had a few hospital visits. As Andy had to go with me we left Charlotte in charge of the shop and she coped brilliantly.

We had the same sort of humour and got on really well and she could read me. For instance if we had a difficult customer and I couldn't cope with them then I just looked at her and she took over. That gave me a break and then I could step in and help later on if need be. Another talent she had was that she could sense that a customer wouldn't look after a costume and steer them towards one that I was not so proud of, if you know what I mean. I also got this feeling with customers and I thought that I was being paranoid.

This proved that I wasn't!

Char has been like a second daughter to me, thank you Jackie for letting me 'borrow' her. She went to University in September 2005 and her sister Sasha took over the helm!

Sasha is a free spirit with a great sense of humour and she proved to be an asset on the days that I felt really bad. She cheered me up and loved everything about fancy dress. I had to teach her quickly, but she was a fast learner and she had already been helping Charlotte on our busy days.

As well as the girls helping me, my family have always been supportive. My Dad by transporting me all over the place. If I needed any material he and my step Mum Josie would take me to buy it. We have been everywhere to buy stuff! Josie also ironed for me until she became too poorly with the big C (she is now in remission, thank God) and it left a big gap in my life. That sounds selfish but it's not meant to be. We just got into a routine and used to put music on and sing, (in a fashion), whilst I was washing and she was ironing. Music is great to get through those tedious jobs!

Nearly everybody, friends and family have done some fancy dress ironing! It's a thankless task, but I thought the costumes always looked better; maybe I was/am too fussy. Joanne my sister is a dyspraxic and likes to help and she was a great help at Galas and fetes. She was a 'watcher' which was a very important job as we had a lot of items pinched. It was amazing how much stock we lost this way!

My most loyal assistant is my hubby Andy who has always been there for me and without whom I couldn't have strived to be 'normal'. Well as normal as normal can be!

14   *The Changing Room & Strange Requests*

WITHOUT CUSTOMERS I wouldn't have had a business, simple as that. Throughout the 16 years of running the shop I have made some good friends and in any business you have to look after your regulars. They brought in new customers and made my life easier.

There have been lots of laughs along the way and some strange customers……..

Once people went into the changing room and that curtain was drawn around them they used to start telling me all their problems! Some of them were quite gross, I mean get a life! I used to get quite embarrassed and was pleased that the curtain was there to stop the customer seeing me pulling faces. I often didn't know what to say, I just oohed and ahhed in the right places.

A lot of women were a bit nervous about me looking at their body to size them up and most are a mixture of two sizes. So I used to close the curtains and say; 'Don't worry, I'm not into women!' This usually did the trick and they relaxed, but on a few occasions a woman would reply; 'Shame!' I couldn't believe it, me getting chatted up by a woman, they must be blind!

I've seen enough bodies to fill a battleship, every size, every shape. Some of them thought they were a God or a Goddess and really loved themselves. They would stand in the changing room and prance and preen in front of the mirror. Some of these customers were really awful, in looks as well as in personality; it took all my patience not to say anything rude to them. One of them reduced me to tears as she tore shreds off me after an hour of undivided attention. It took a long while to get my confidence back as it's never been high. A good job I have a great husband and friends.

One day this large plain looking woman charged into the shop and announced; 'I need a shag tonight, what have you got that will fit me?' I was shocked, stuck for words (this doesn't happen very often!) and I just stared at her. I was old enough to be her mother, had she no pride? I had just finished making a large Xena and got her into the changing room fast, so she didn't upset any of the other customers. It looked brilliant on her and she loved it. One of my quickest hires. When she brought the outfit back she said; 'Oh that was fantastic! I pulled a great guy and we shagged all night on my kitchen table. The noise the costume made (I had sewn loads of metal buttons and discs on it) was brill, it sounded like little cymbals!' I thought plerrrrrease, toooo much information; I do not want that thought all day! Needless to say Xena went in the washer three times as every time I took it out, I couldn't touch it, and so I put it back in again!

The first time that I had a deep breather on the phone he asked if I sold rubber wear! I was really shocked! After a few of these strange requests I became accustomed to them and learned to laugh them off.

For at least two years we had regular phone calls from this man that we nicknamed 'the Vicar'. The reason for this was he sounded just like my Uncle Peter who was a vicar and had a lovely, quietly spoken voice.

That's where the similarity ended! This man was really kinky. He always asked if I had any punk gear and was it leather or P.V.C. and did I have a t-shirt with the nipples exposed. Also did I sell nipple chains?

Honestly, do I look as if I sell nipple chains? I only have one tattoo and I was a big baby after having that one done! (a 40 year old thing).

He once phoned about putting a play on and what was my hire charge for a lot of costumes. I spent ages on the phone with him, but he didn't turn up. Andy said he must like my deep voice and he just wanted to keep me talking to him! Then after a while he actually came into the shop and I didn't realize that it was him. It suddenly came to me and I thought; 'Oh no, it's the Vicar, what am I going to do? So I just kept calm and then surprise, surprise, what did he want to try on.....a punk! He went into the changing room with the costume and after a lot of grunts he went quiet. I intrepidly asked if he was alright and was dreading opening the curtains. When I did he was trying to take his photo through the mirror! He had also put some weird make-up on and I just stood there agog. He looked at me as if this was the norm and asked; 'Would you like your photo taking with me this feels sooooooooo sexy! I turned tail and ran downstairs calling for Andy, who took over and asked him to politely leave. We never heard from him again, thank goodness!

I will always remember the busy Christmas when this couple walked in. Now, this pair were a very pretty couple, him with long blonde hair & sunglasses and her with long black hair & sunglasses. They both wore very long leather coats and looked like something off the matrix. I did my sales pitch and invited them to look through the fancy dress books. When the changing room became free I took them upstairs and found their costumes for them. I asked if they were ok and they replied; 'Yes thank you very much'. So I went and stood on the stairs and started helping someone else.   After a while I called upstairs to see if they were alright and did they need any help. No reply.

Then we heard funny noises coming from the changing room. A hush fell on the whole shop. You could have heard a pin drop if it wasn't for the grunts coming from upstairs.

This couple were actually bonking in my changing room and everyone was listening! I didn't know what to do, so I went downstairs and waited behind the desk. After what seemed like an eternity they came downstairs as if nothing had happened and said; 'We've changed our minds thank you', then walked out of the shop. Well, then everyone in the shop starting clapping and cheering! It was so funny. I mean I've heard of having fantasies in cemeteries and on the top of a double decker bus, but in a changing room?

I ask you, it takes all sorts to make a world, but sometimes do you ever wonder?

15   *Photographing & Videoing*

I STARTED OFF displaying photographs of the fancy dress on a type of carousel photo unit in the shop. As I made more costumes this became rather full so I needed to do something different and better. I had used friends and family for models and it made it easier by having a photographer as a husband. Andy and I sat and talked and we decided to keep taking the photos but make them bigger and put them in photograph albums which we stacked on the floor in front of a display shelf.

Customers saw these as soon as they came into the shop and were easy to look at. This worked well, but it took a lot of work keeping them looking good as the books would get mistreated. The more costumes I made meant more books and I ended up with 15 books and on a lot of the pages we had 2 photos or more.

Whenever a friend came to see me, I would grab them for a photo shoot, no wonder they didn't come very often! Actually some of them loved it and were always phoning me up to see if I had made another costume. My daughter and my assistants were good models as they were slim and young and they were brilliant. I used all shapes and ages for models. One day a customer tried on a new costume and asked me to take her photo, so I used my Polaroid camera and then I thought; 'Hang on; we could use customers photos in the books!' So we did this and had some really funny ones!

When I redid or changed a costume I had to take another photo of it. I was always adding costumes to the books and I changed the books for new ones once or twice a year. It was a good job that I bought the photo albums wholesale.

The books were ok, but we needed something else to keep peoples attention if I was busy with another customer so we bought a small combi television/video recorder. Then we asked friends and family if they would dress up in the costumes while we videoed them. They and lots more agreed, which surprised me! Nearly everyone who saw the video playing in the shop wanted to be in it! We used our studio and supplied wine which was an essential ingredient if you want happy relaxed people. I didn't drink any as half a glass and I'm solid gone! I had already worked out which costumes we were going to video and had written them down. This worked well and we did very short amateurish sketches. We did a couple of video sessions a year which took all evening to do 15 minutes of tape, but we didn't half have some fun! Goodness knows what some of the customers thought of it, but some of them chuckled so it couldn't have been that bad. The only thing was that we were always short of slimmish men for models as they seemed to be terribly shy. I suppose the 'Oh sod it, I don't care' attitude comes to us all with age!

The tape would wear out as it was played over and over again, so we had to re-edit it quite often. Also sometimes if a costume no longer existed, (like Gary Glitter, what a moron!) or I updated a costume they had to be edited out which was time consuming but a good result. We ended up buying three combi TV's over the years!

After a couple of years though, I got fed up with hearing my voice droning on in the background. The bit where I said; 'when will we three meet again' in a crackly voice really, really got on my nerves! So we put our heads together again and decided to use film tracks.

This worked well, but took a lot of putting together; don't forget this was before the digital revolution. I quite like choreographing it and will always remember Andy dressed as Dart Vade and Jono (Emma's fella) dressed as a Jedi Knight.

When the Star Wars theme started they went at it hammer and tongue with their light sabres as if they were really battling for the

Empire! Our twin grandsons who were about 4 years old then and were watching, shouted; 'Oh no, don't kill Granddad!' Realism or what?

When digital came in it made it easier for me to print photos out and also we did quite large ones which looked very good hanging up high in the shop.

I could go on about all the photos and the videoing and bore you to tears, let's just say it was hilarious, hard work and great fun, but I will tell you about the last session that we did. Andy had always wanted to do a Monty Python sketch and he loved the lumberjack song. So he dressed in the Mountie outfit and the girls wore saucy Red Indian outfits. I'm a lumberjack started playing and Andy (he loves singing and being a fool), started miming it and literally threw himself into the part. It was brilliant! We thought that we would be a bit naughty so we stopped the video and Andy changed into the large PVC French maid which fitted where it touched and then we started filming again. He just stood there with his feather duster looking like a transvestite gone wrong and we all shouted; 'Oh No!', then threw cushions at him! When people watched this they couldn't believe that Andy would dress up like this and thought that I had made him do it! Honestly, I just suggested it and he went along with it. Good laugh though!

At the same time Charlotte and Kirsti dressed up in the 70's 'pimps'(huggy bear from Starsky and Hutch) and Rob, Char's fella, as Rod Stewart. We played; 'Do you think I'm sexy' and all three of them went into overdrive. The girls had stuffed socks down the front of their trousers and strutted their stuff for all that it was worth! Half way through the song we stopped videoing and put balloons down the back of Rob's trousers. Those of you old enough to remember Kenny Everet will know this sketch. Laugh, we were rolling on the floor! You could hear us on the video!

When there were children in the shop I had to turn the video off if this was on. It was hilarious and I miss those barmy nights.

Once I was upstairs helping a customer and Charlotte was showing another one of the books. Now there is a photo of me as a belly dancer and I didn't think I looked too bad in it as I was thinner then (still 16 stones, but my tummy was flat). As my health got worse I got bigger and by the time I closed the shop I was nearly 20 stones! Anyway this woman looked at the photo and said; 'She's fat isn't she?' I thought charming and I looked over the banister and retorted; 'I am cuddly not fat and what you see is what you get!' Enough said and everyone cheered in the shop.

Go on, laugh, you'll live longer, I have!

16   *the Busiest Time of the Year*

I USED TO both detest and relish New Year week. This was the week following Boxing Day and finishing on the 31st. It was pure GRIND.   Work, smile, work, smile, grovel and count to ten a lot of times (but only with the annoying customers). Its great when the money comes in and after paying the girls that week, what was left was my main yearly wage. We opened at 10am and we didn't close until sometimes nearly 9pm. We worked straight through and kept going on coffee and sandwiches which Andy would make and put in your hand so you ate them! That was the money week and if you didn't take it, then you were doing something terribly wrong.

You had to be there all the time but at least I could sleep until 8am, which is how I got through the week, plus pain killers.

I loved the regulars; most of them were so amenable and really easy to get along with. They used to come in, look through the fancy dress books, have a chat and choose what they wanted. Simple, but they weren't all like this. Some of them could see that we were really, really busy but all that mattered to them was themselves. They would rant about a costume that was already booked and could we phone up that customer and ask if they had changed their minds as they wanted it! Are you real? Get out of my shop! Thank goodness I didn't get too many selfish people in.

One of my regular groups of people used to do a theme each New Year and a few years ago they came into the shop in October. They would book early to get what they wanted. Anyway one of the women said; 'Right Pen, I want to be Friar Tuck!' She was about the same size as me (5ft 8in and cuddly) and I laughed; 'Why Friar Tuck?' She grinned; 'I know that it will fit me and the best of all I can carry a box of wine around all night with no questions asked!' Fair enough!

Batman and the super hero costumes were always booked before the last week and I would have loved to hang a sign outside the shop saying; No Batman's or Jedi's left!

So there were a lot of blokes who had to rethink their costumes. Cowboys and Pirates were good macho costumes and I would do them proud. The funny thing was that these macho men wanted frilly pirate shirts! I always put loads of accessories with my costumes as boys will be boys and what's a pirate without a sword & hook? Captain hook was my favourite and he was usually booked out fairly early

Andy was always being asked to be Santa at Christmas for the local school and I think he is looking more and more like him!

The Christmas week was not as intense but still busy. It was the same routine. Work, close the shop, eat and rest then wash the smelly fancy dress which had been tried on by people who don't believe in soap. Also the changing area had to be tidied every night.

So it was always midnight before we got to bed.

I LOVE Christmas! It is and always will be a magical time for children and adults who care to make it so. Life is what you make it to be. We always had Christmas day off and a few days before this we would start to clear away the fancy dress from the sitting room. This included the ironing board which was ALWAYS up.

I lived by this golden rule; on Christmas Eve and Day the sitting room was ours and we had to have at least one room clear of shop stuff or else I would have gone mad! Even so, we worked Christmas Eve until 4pm and after then customers would knock on the back door to return their costumes that they had worn at work that day. These would be washed straight away and hung in the shop which now had the wood burner lit (which was usually buried under stock).

We would have to listen out for the washer and dryer, but at least for two wonderful days we had a nearly 'normal' life!

In fact we moved the sewing table out of the sitting room on the 1st December because I loved Christmas so much and against Andy's moanings I wanted the tree up then. The fireplace was decorated and by the time we finished it looked like Santa's grotto (still does!), but it was worth all the time and effort. Every time I went into the sitting room, particularly after a difficult customer, I felt happy and peaceful. After a few choice words to no one in particular, I would look around and say; 'Sod 'em!' The world does not revolve around them and I must never, ever turn into a demanding bitchy woman. I have my moments, mind you, just like everyone else but these are short lived.

When I could drink alcohol without getting drunk on half a glass of wine, I would walk into the sitting room after a stressful customer and Andy would be standing there with a 'happy coffee' (coffee and whiskey). Later on it was coffee and a cuddle, but it still did the trick.

Going back to New Year's week. It was great when a customer used to come in, get what they wanted, paid with no complains and then said; 'Thank you'. Lovely! It was also a great feeling when we had a queue of people waiting outside the shop because we were so busy and there wasn't any room for them inside. I used to swell with pride and think; 'this is MINE, I've made it like it is and nobody can alter that. It will be sad to finish, it's my life, my baby, but at least I made it my way'.

By New Years Eve night we were all jiggered, knackered, call it what you like. There was no greater feeling than spreading £2,000 plus of my hard earned money out and knowing that you've made it with your own blood sweat and tears (metaphorically speaking). Every year I usually bought something that we needed. The first year we bought our bedroom wardrobes and its great to look at those now and think; 'I bought those with my first fancy dress wages!'

17   *Fancy Dress Ruled My Life!*

THE FANCY DRESS BUSINESS devours you, lock stock and barrel! I ate, slept and dreamt it for 16 years. People used to think because I lived next to the shop that I was on call for every hour of the day even on Christmas day when they would knock on the door and ask me to sell them batteries. After a few months of being open we bought an answering machine and had on it; sorry, we are closed at the moment, but please leave a message and I'll get back to you as soon as possible. I changed this message quite often. Now, we had a phone in the shop and one in the sitting room with an answer machine, so if friends or family phoned we could hear them shouting; 'It's me, pick up the phone!' It's amazing how many me's we knew! We all do this, but sometimes a customer would do it and I would pick up thinking that it was a friend and then find out it was someone asking me to open up again. The amount of people who didn't really leave a message but carried on talking to a person in the same room as them, usually saying this; 'They're f-----g closed again!', was unbelievable. Yes, of course we were closed on Sundays, (open Oct to Dec), and at night past 9pm! Honestly! Sometimes we tried to have a life.

We did up to nine washes a day and had two washing machines and we were always listening out to empty and refill the washer and tumble dryer. This became an automatic reaction. As I have already said, the sitting room wasn't mine as it was always full of fancy dress repairs, drying or ironing. The ironing board was always up and we got through two irons a year as they couldn't cope with all the work.

The worst time for washing was when the New Year fancy dress was returned. We had a system without which we couldn't have coped. Before anything was returned we would light scented candles and joss sticks to mask the smell of cigarettes that would stink the sitting room out. Then we covered the armchairs with black bags so we could empty the costume bags onto them. They would be sorted out into colours and bagged up. Accessories would be put on one side to be hand washed later. The bags were stacked up in the darkroom. Over the next few weeks we would work our way through the mound of washing bags, believe it or not there was loads of black items in the costumes. So basically I washed in 'colours', a bag at a time. It was dismal having a lot of black washing hanging to dry around you so I tried to wash different colours. Each night I washed the accessories and we would put them away.

Sometimes it took more than four weeks to wash all the New Year costumes. It was very common at this time of the year for us to run out of clean undies!

My family helped me get through all the ironing and we had two ironing boards up to tackle it all. The repairs were done in between all this; in fact repairs were non-stop, always ongoing.

In February when it was all done we would close the shop and disappear for a week's holiday which coincided with our wedding anniversary. I loved these breaks and would come back all refreshed and full of new ideas.

Fancy Dress is and will always be, in my blood and I see possibilities for costumes everywhere. This suits my hyperactive mind and I can't settle for long (though since being retired I find this easier to do!). It's not in my nature to just sit and watch the TV. I am usually doing something else such as a crossword. (Nowadays I write this book!) When I had the shop I did the books at night and sorted out the next order.

There was always such a lot to do and because I have a short term memory I had a notebook (still have) nearby with a list of 'jobs' on it. This was vital whilst running the shop. It reminded of my own personnel 'jobs' to do so I was organised, which I desperately needed to be.

Our gardening and things like decorating the house tended to be left in favour of the shop. I was always tired and my house hadn't been properly decorated in years.

I can remember the year when our twin grandsons were born and Kirsti was still living with us. They arrived a bit earlier than expected and in between hospital visits and running the shop, we painted the sitting room. The thing was that I painted around the picture frames and cupboards and nobody noticed until we have cable television put in and we had to move the furniture. Well, that back wall looked like a chess board and was my face red!

Every time we had some 'us time' something else cropped up either to do with the shop or the village, (we are in a few village groups). Do you know what I missed the most? Christmas Shopping! Why, you ask? Well for years I had to shop out of a catalogue and the reason?.....time.

What with longer working hours, weekend opening and evening bookings I didn't have time to turn around. I needed the wages and I had to work, like most people, but the bills and the assistant's wages came first before paying me.

Anyway back to Christmas. I missed the build up to it and all the excitement that went with it. Of course I got a lot of Christmas spirit through the customers and the T.V., but nothing beats going out and seeing the lights and drinking in the atmosphere.

The pride that I got from people hiring out my costumes made up for some of what I missed out on. That is until my body couldn't keep up with my mind.

I had to change my lifestyle.

Saying this, we've had some fun times; where else could you dress up for work? Andy & I love and try to embrace life, but during the last year of opening my memory became worse.

This was because of a mixture of all the fits and falls that I have had and the side effects of my epilepsy tablets. My specialist kept telling me to finish work.

It was really embarrassing forgetting customer's names and what costume that they had booked. Also I was having trouble breathing and had chest pains. I couldn't run up the stairs with an arm full of outfits without clutching my chest because of the pain. I would often sit on the top step to get my breath.

Andy had bought me a bike the year before and we tried to go out on short 'bike' rides (Andy in his electric wheelchair) around the village. It was great to get out and escape!

I ended up collapsing whilst biking up a hill. I woke up in hospital and was told it was a small heart attack and they told me to stop riding my bike.

So I ended up going to a heart specialist and after a few tests he put me on heart tablets and aspirin. I wasn't over eating and my weight soared up to 19 and a half stones!

I was in a turmoil. I needed to exercise to lose weight, but I was told to rest!

I have never been a big eater so we reckoned my weight problem was due to all the steroids in my tablets. Including vitamins I was on 12 tablets plus a day.

My assistants 'carried' me, they became my memory and made me sit down more.

I'm sure some of the customers thought I was batty, (many of my friends think I have always been so!) and I realized that I couldn't go on, I had to give up.

18   *My Last Christmas & New Year*

MY LAST CHRISTMAS and New Year was awful because I kept bursting into tears all the time! All I could think was; 'I'm only 50 years old and I have to give work. I'm a failure'. Of course this was utter tosh, but that's me all over.

It was both a great time and a sad time as this was my last ever, ever, ever Christmas and New Year in my shop.

We have always had fun times and a good laugh in between the hard work and the 'difficult' customers. This year was a little different as the Internet had crept into my life with a vengeance. People were spending large amounts of money with them on outfits that left nothing to the imagination, but they were still coming to me for accessories. I couldn't believe how much they spent on an outfit, when they could have hired a complete one off me and had change.

It was also exhausting as two of my helpers were at University and they didn't come home until just before Christmas Day. So it was just me and Andy in the week and Sasha at the weekends. Andy was in constant pain with his leg. He had acupuncture every two weeks which only lasted for one week and because he was on his feet more by helping me he was on pain killers. I was having problems getting my breath and I was having more fits, so I was on 1,000mg of tegretol a day instead of 800mg which left me feeling sick and a bit dozy. I was told to take an extra tegretol on bad days by my doctor.

I couldn't have coped without Andy as that year we worked straight through for 13 days until Christmas Eve.

We were invited out on Christmas Eve by our friends Rachel and Paul. For the past few years we have always declined, but this year Andy said; 'Sod it, yes please!' I was surprised and knew we would be doing the fancy dress laundry when we got back, but looked forward to going out for a few hours. So feeling a bit like zombies we walked down our road. It was lovely getting out in the fresh air. I stopped on the corner and Andy asked me what the matter was. I replied; 'nothing', but it had just struck me that I hadn't even had time to come out and look at the Christmas lights on the peoples houses. It was at his moment that I realised that I hadn't had a 'proper' Christmas for the past 16 years. Oh sure, I had a lovely Christmas day with the family, but I never really had the time to relax and enjoy it properly. Even our friends stopped asking us to their Christmas & New Year parties. Thanks goodness Rachel never gave up!

It was at this point standing at the bottom of our street that I knew that I needed to close, the business was killing me, I needed a life.

After a lovely Christmas Eve and Day, Kirsti and I spent our last Boxing Day ever, ironing. Thank goodness for that, it will be great to 'lounge' on Boxing Day!

As we were closing we printed out small leaflets saying; 'Sorry, due to ill health Pens Fancy Dress will be closing for good on Friday February 17th 2006'. Also there was a date for the Auction. We had a giant sign up in the shop and in the display windows. There was a mixed reaction from the customers from these. Most of them were lovely and said that they would miss me.

A lot of them came in on the last week with friends and family to buy stock that they might need in the future and I gave them a good deal on it.   For the past few years Andy & I used to dress up for a themed personal Christmas card that we gave to friends and family. We usually did this in November and we suddenly realised that we would never have this wealth of costumes to choose from again! We've done all sorts; Elves, Andy as Santa and me as Rudolph and this year (2005) we decided to be a Christmas tree and a Christmas cracker and go out with a bang! Not literally.

Anyway back to work…….

New Year week was always a hard slog and this one was of no exception. The days started up slowly and then boom, we were packed out until nearly 8pm every night. Luckily I had a lot of helpers and Andy worked in the background feeding us and making hot drinks. Every night I collapsed on the settee for a few 'winks' and then later he helped me tidy the shop. Also I had the bookings to go through.

There was one thing that was worrying me this year and what if the costumes weren't returned seeing as we were closing? I needn't have worried as they all came back on time and a few of the customers asked if they could buy them. I had to turn them down as they were already numbered for the auction, but now I wish I sold it to them. Learn from me, if a customer gives you a good price then sell it to them! Mind you a lot of the offers were silly, like £5,000 for all 700 costumes. So stick to your guns. After New Year when all the costumes were returned, I stood in the sitting room surrounded by smelly, dirty outfits and it was wonderful to think; 'Never again!'

19   *The Auction, Before, During & After*

I T HAS TAKEN OVER A YEAR since closing the shop to write this chapter. It is now April 2007 and I can now cope with looking at the fancy dress books and auction lists without bursting into tears. I suppose I am the emotional type.

From September 2005 I had to organise the closing of my business. First of all I telephoned the Auctioneers and they came to see me. All 700 of my fancy dress costumes were going to Auction in April 2006 and I had to make a detailed category list. This was hard going and heart breaking to do. I kept crying for no reason at all and I felt so depressed. I was actually going to finish the shop, this was final.

It suddenly hit home, I was no longer going to be self employed with my own business which is something I am proud of, but I was going to be unemployed and disabled. I know that I am an epileptic and now have some sort of heart problem, but I have always thought of myself as 'normal with a few problems'.

The customer's reaction to me closing was mixed. I was amazed at some of them who said; 'Oh, no now what am I going to do?' Selfish or what? I sarcastically replied, 'Ok, I'll just wait until the business gives me a wooden overcoat then!'

Most of them though were great and I thank them for their concern. The thing is that I look quite healthy, if you don't look at me for too long! Underneath though I feel awful and just want to curl up under a blanket. This wasn't always possible with running a busy fancy dress shop, so I didn't often get the chance to rest and recoup.

Getting back to the category list, which proved to be a mammoth task? I did it alphabetically and went through all the costumes making sure that each one had the right accessories. Something that I wish I hadn't been so fastidious about.

In January 2006 after the New Year costumes had been washed, ironed and repaired I put large cards with numbers on each one of them. This took ages, every minute of the day and half the night was spent 'doing the list'. I had to do this on my own as I was the only one who knew what went with what and Andy would say; 'Come on love finish for the night and sit down' I would reply ; 'When I've finished the P's' or something like that, sounds funny now!

We also had to find space to hang all the costumes in order and they took up more room because of all the accessories hanging from them. We put them in the Garage (Studio) on make shift rails out of tripods and poles and kept some heating on so they wouldn't go damp. The rails were so close that we couldn't get between them which didn't help when we found a missing item.

As I was numbering up I was thinking; 'these will be in a different shop soon and I hope they look after them' Sad I know, but I didn't want to let them go.

Whilst sorting them out I couldn't believe all the dust! Some rooms in our house hadn't seen daylight in years and it was hard work emptying and cleaning them. I was sneezing non stop. I'm not saying my costumes were dusty; it was the moving of them that caused a lot of it.

The last week of opening was the worst, I was so down. Andy had cleared both the display windows and had put blinds up in them which made it feel cosier. This helped as I got through the week by imagining two armchairs in front of the fire and it being MY room. Thank goodness for me being able to day dream!

My son, his partner and children came up from London to help and support me and my daughter, her partner and children were with me, so I had my whole family around me. Andy hardly left my side, he is my rock and he and my family are my reason for living and battling on.

I spent the last day of opening in a haze. I had put on wine and nibbles and all through the day customers and friends came in to say god luck with the future. The Rose wine was lovely; maybe that's why I was in a haze! (Only sips, honest!) On This day, the 17th February was our 31st wedding anniversary and I realised that I had spent half our married life in the shop.

The next day was Andy's birthday and we spent the whole day clearing the shop. He said it was a great day as he had got me back and he was going to make sure that I was staying around for a lot longer! Kirsti, Ross and their families worked like Trojans and the shop was quickly cleared. I just kept packing boxes and they were taken off me and stored away. When all the shelves were taken down we just stood and stared at the walls. There were loads of lines of varnish and masses of raw plugs, hooks & nails all over them.

I remember going into the sitting room and my youngest grandson, Jonathan looked at me and said; 'Mamma, it's snowing dust!' Sure enough with the sun shining through the window it looked like dusty snow.

I spent the first week of closing feeling really depressed. I couldn't even go outside and look at the front of the house as it looked lost, weird, just a normal house again.

The second week was better as I realised that I could walk down to the local shop or around the village without worrying about getting back to the shop.

I was still sorting and numbering costumes so that kept me busy.

We went into Nottingham and I was so used to looking for fancy dress material etc that I felt lost and I had to go and buy some buttons to Andy's great amusement!

Sunday 2nd April, oh what a day! We started bringing costumes down from the upper 'shop' room to the lower as we wanted them downstairs to make it easier for moving them out. It was hard work as we had to move two large pine rails which had been up there for 13 years. Of course we ran out of room quite quickly as we hadn't any hooks etc in the walls to hang costumes on. You should have seen it! There were costumes over doors in the hallway, in fact everywhere.

We finished at about 4pm when disaster struck, one of the pine rails snapped with all the weight and the whole lot tipped forward and smashed into the 'shop' glass front door. We both rushed into the room and couldn't believe our eyes! The door is double glazed and there was a hole about the size of an egg with cracks going from it. Luckily it only broke the inside pane which had a notice on and broke the impact. Kirsti, who lives across the road, heard the noise and came running over. Very quickly all of us grabbed the costumes off the rail and piled them on the settee or the pole would have gone straight through the door. So we ended up hanging them from the sitting room ceiling beams on long canes.

These took most of them and the rest hung anywhere we had space.

The studio was full of 300 costumes and the downstairs 'shop' room had 300, so we had 100 in the sitting room and hallway.

This worked ok until about 7.30pm when the canes gave an almighty crack and the whole lot fell down! By this time we had had enough, but we put in loads of hooks in the beams and transferred the costumes to these which took ages. We were both shattered and it was like sitting in a forest so we called it a day.

Monday the 3rd April is one day that I would like to forget about! It started off quite smoothly with our friends and families arriving in their cars which we loaded up with costumes. Kirsti and I went with my Dad to the Auction rooms were about 20 miles from us, so it was a long round trip. Andy stayed at home to help load up cars with the rest of the costumes. Everyone who helped on this day were brilliant, some of them even declined the petrol money we gave them.

It's great to have friends and family like this.

On arrival at the Auction rooms I was shown where the costumes were being hung. I was devastated as it was a 'warehouse' room with a dusty concrete floor and two loading bays, so it was freezing! I couldn't believe it, after all the months of heating the studio and shop to keep the costumes from going damp; here was a place like the Antarctic, with dust! Kirsti looked at me, gave me a cuddle and said; 'Come on Mum, they won't be here long, lets unload'. So we set too.

It was an organised bedlam. We ran out of rails as five of the smaller ones just collapsed and broke. I had no choice but to buy ten new rails from nearby shop fitters, costing me £300. This meant I could spread the costumes out and I recouped some of the money by selling them in the Auction, but it was an expense that I hadn't bargained for.

Andy arrived and Kirsti had to leave, so Andy and I spent all day sorting the fancy dress out into numeral order. It was a nightmare! We also did this on Tuesday & Wednesday.

Dad ferried us around and each night we came home, drank a gallon of tea with painkillers, had a 'sad' meal (frozen dinner), soaked in the bath and were in bed by 9pm. It was agonizing. Andy put acupuncture needles in his leg every night to keep the pain at bay, he was wonderful. I was having several petits every day because of the stress but I had to keep pushing myself on.

The Auctioneers were amazed at our hard work and said we were the most organised customers that they had had. We took this to mean; 'Thanks because we haven't had to pay someone to sort this lot out we will give you discount'. No chance.

On Thursday and Friday we didn't go and rested up. The Auctioneers asked us to go in on Saturday afternoon to spread the rails out as there would be more room. We had never seen all our costumes together and were flabbergasted. How had our poor floors managed to take the weight?

Our 'shop rooms' now echoed!

I couldn't sleep, my nerves were shot. I was so worried that they wouldn't sell.

Monday 10th April was viewing day and we went in with the portable TV, video and fancy dress books. I was dreading it. There were people looking at MY costumes and I didn't like it one bit. I smiled, bit my lip, all I wanted to do was to gather them all up and run home with them!

Quite a few people turned up and there weren't many awful comments I kept going and standing outside, it was torture. What surprised me though was the distance some people had come. Some had come from Wales and were staying in a hotel, for my costumes!

That night I walked the boards, I couldn't sleep.

Tuesday 11th April 2006. D day. I forced myself to smile and got on with it, even though it felt like my world was falling through a big black hole.

Some of my costumes went so cheaply that I kept going to the loo and had a cry. I couldn't cope, but I had to. I didn't want to have a fit in front of all these people.

There were some good moments like when my lion went for £105! Also one of my customers who had hired the American Officer off me was there and he bought it. That cheered me up as it was going to someone who would look after it.

All in all most of the costumes went for a good price, the rest I don't want to think about.

The nice thing about the day was that the buyers kept coming up to me and asking if I was the seller. Thinking that they were going to moan at me, I just nodded my head, but they were lovely. Most of them said the costumes were great and made with love and care. I was honoured with this and the greatest compliment I could have had from another Fancy dress owner. One woman had travelled all the way from Cornwall and asked for my address so that she could send me photos of her shop. I declined and said politely no thank you. I was grateful she had bought them, but I wasn't coping that well letting them go. She understood and I hope they brought her good luck.

A couple of buyers asked if I was alright as I looked distraught. They couldn't believe that I was selling up. They were lovely people and I told them I was an epileptic and had to give up because of health problems. I tried not to think too much about it or else I would have cracked up. I even got asked my phone number but in my haze I gave them the shop one which no longer exists.

It was a long heartbreaking day and I was glad when I left the Auction rooms for the last time. I never want to go there again, too many memories.

The proceeds went to pay off our mortgage and decorate some of the house. So as they say; C'est la vie!

I didn't get as much for my costumes as I hoped for, but as my Gran always told me; never cry over spilt milk. I was starting a new life.

It was an awful feeling, in fact I had a break down and it took me months to get over it. I threw myself into decorating the shop rooms and they look so bright! Every time I went in the spare room to sort out the stock and albums, I burst into tears, so I left that job until later. Writing this book has helped as I didn't realise how much time and effort that I had spent in/on the shop. It made me think how lucky I was now being able to go out on a walk with my grandchildren and simple things like being able to sit and watch and film all the way through instead of sewing or falling asleep! Christmas 2006 was brilliant as I went Christmas shopping and lost myself in the great atmosphere with carols being sung and people being so happy. I went to Church and watched the grandchildren in their Christmas play and we even had a Christmas Party! Our house was packed with friends and family.

We both helped on the Sleigh run, Andy as Santa and me an Elf (a big one!) which was great fun. I even joined Felley Players our local drama group although I am not that good and my memory is rubbish, but it's good fun and filled a bit of the void in my life. Working kept me going, so I have had to find other things to feed my hyper active brain, even though my body is trailing behind!

On Boxing Day we lounged, which was a strange feeling, I kept thinking that I should be doing something else. In fact we lounged nearly all week, good job we are surrounded by some wonderful countryside to help walk the weight off! If I feel down this is a great healer just to sit at the top of a hilly field and soak in nature. It's good to be alive!

On reflection over the 16 years of having the shop I enriched my life with meeting all these colourful characters and I have done something that I have always wanted to do.

Ok, I have a disability, but that doesn't and never has stopped me completely. I loved my job and I miss a lot about it, but I have another life and I am content!

My life has turned around in the two years of finishing the shop. It is more peaceful, well sometimes! After a series of heart tests the specialist realised that it was my lungs that were the problem not my heart. So I came off the heart tablets and started losing weight. Then I went through more tests on my lungs and I have been diagnosed with emphysema. This was most probably caused by all the smelly costumes and all the sprays I used to get them clean.

So, now I am on inhalers and don't use or go near toxic cleaners and smokers. My heart attack was caused by stress and not being able to breathe properly.

I am a great believer in natural healants, like cinnamon sticks in my coffee to help my lungs and every 3 weeks I go to my friend Pauline who is a holistic therapist and gives me a full body massage. This helps the pain caused by all my falls and the Arthritis I now have in all my joints.

I have lost two stones over the past two years, but if I have to go on a weeks steroids for my lungs I can put a stone back on in a week! This year I have been lucky.

I still have fits; I had a bad fall not long ago, but am ok now. I got worried about being in a play, silly me, so am having a rest from the drama group for a while.

That's my life, good days and bad days! I miss going on long walks and running, but I have started swimming again. If you can call it swimming, a length then resting for your lungs to catch up!

Funnily enough I miss alcohol as I can't cope with it. I am wappy enough without it!

Ok, I get upset and cross when I can't do things and get down, but never, ever do what I did once and that was to flush all my tablets down the loo because I wanted to be normal. I ended up in hospital, it was a near one!

I am still here and feel very lucky.

.o0o.

LOOKING GLASS COLLECTION

There, with the Grace of God , would go - I a collection of real life stories of ordinary folk in different surroundings, which reveal the extraordinary resilience and range of characteristics of the human personality.

Gloucester Editions   - (rrp £6-95)

'Shrink in the Clink' by Michael Haslam   978-1-904494-99-7
A revealing, eye-opening account of an inmate serving time in a modern H.M. Prison.

'My Life in Mental Chains' by Ruth Hartman 978-1-904494-98-0
Her Obsessive Compulsive Disorder (OCD) began gradually, but it became a frightening memory that has been seared into her mind with a painful brand.

'Class War' by Eric R. Brady   978-1-904494-84-3
Adolf Hitler's war machine could not defeat these London school children in this thrilling true life story of young blood, sweat, toil and tears.

'The Enemy Within' by Colin Biggs   978-1-904494-78-2
An heroic battle against the dreaded disease Multiple Sclerosis by a trained firefighter who fought his illness with true courage!

'Though My Eyes' by Vendon Wright   978-1-904494-86-7
The story of a Black Belt Master of Taekwondo who lost his sight but gained on in-sight.

'Nine Lives' by Colin Biggs   978-1-904494-95-9
Nine moving stories how nine incredible people coped with losing their limbs.

'Jasmine' by Jasmine Maria Hill   978-1-904494-94-2
The story of the girl from a Children's Home, beautifully told through this collection of poems by the author.

Salisbury Editions - (rrp £4-95)

'Nurse, Nurse!' by Nurse Lucy Samuels   978-1-904494-58-4
The amusing experiences of a dedicated and caring NHS nurse and her patients in hospital.

'Present, Miss!' by Frances Lea-Riley   978-1-904494-71-3
An inspiring and moving story of a successful teacher, for all those who are thinking about joining this worthwhile profession.

'A Teacher's Depression' by Ian Mallon   978-1-904494-63-8
The personal experiences of a dedicated and caring school teacher coping with work-related stress.

'What's In A Gamble!' by Jake Brindell   978-1-904494-44-7
The story of a compulsive gambler, and how he gave it up in 100 agonising days. A lesson for us all.

'Tales out of Church' by the Rev. Andrew Sangster 978-1-904494-11-9
Few of us knew what lurked behind a cassock until this revealing humorous collection of tales opened our eyes.

'No Way Out' by Sheila Brookes   978-1-904494-25-6
For two hours, step inside the shoes of a battered wife and experience her twenty years ordeal.

'After Virgo ...' by Keith Johnston   978-1-904494-04-1
Through this work we can share the pain of one diagnosed as having the dreaded disease... and the hopes and fears in the subsequent treatments.

'Reaching the Light at the End of the Tunnel'
by Linda Rowe   978-1 -902628-63-9
A loving wife's story of how she coped with life and supported her husband as he fought the life threatening illness of leukaemia and won.

'The Frequent Trader' by Bob Tyson   978-1-902628-34-9
The story of UK's most successful investor who, without influence, favour, any inside knowledge or previous experience in share dealing, increased the value of his initial savings 68 times its original value in 13 years!

THE YOUNG ONES

Stories for emerging adults about the wonderful new world they are about to enter is not what they expect ...

'No Cuddles Today' by Jackie Kain   ISBN 978-1-902628-62-2
The moving story of a girl, physically abused in childhood, and how she came to terms with life.

'Broken Wings' by Katherine Munro   ISBN 978-1-902628-65-3
The moving story of a girl, mentally abused in childhood, and how she lost her health but maintained her sanity.

'The Russian Girl's Story' by Jeanne Feasey   ISBN 978-1-902628-61-5
Separated from her parents during the war in Eastern Europe, the toddler is brought up by the peasant couple who found her.   Later, at the age of eleven, she finds her father is a high-ranking Russian official, in this moving, eye-opening account of human warmth and tragedy.

'A Somerset Childhood' by Phyllis Wyatt   ISBN 978-1-902628-36-3
This little girl was poor, but she had a happy childhood in a loving family in a beautiful part of the country. For readers who missed a happy childhood, this childhood is one they can, from within the pages of this book, adopt to fill the gap in themselves.

'Stay? No Way!' by Vivienne Loranger   ISBN 978-1-902628-82-0
When two Australian teenagers run away from their homes, they discover much about the cruel world outside - and much more about their own fickle selves.

****

Bargain Book!
A comprehensive volume of stories published in the
Young Ones series is now available
Simply telephone the Publishers on 01249 720563

****

For more book bargains, visit our website at:
WWW.SUPAMASU.COM